Compliments of *W.B. Saunders Company*

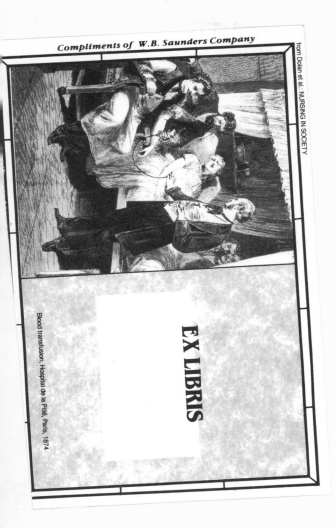

from Dolan et al.: NURSING IN SOCIETY

EX LIBRIS

Blood transfusion, Hospital de la Pitié, Paris, 1874

Ocular
Motility
and
Strabismus

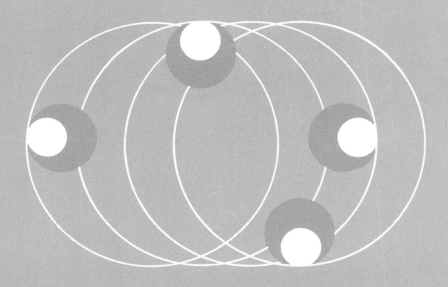

**OCULAR MOTILITY AND STRABISMUS is included
(first section, volume I) in CLINICAL OPHTHALMOLOGY, a four-volume loose-leaf series
edited by Thomas D. Duane, M.D., published by Harper & Row.**

OCULAR MOTILITY AND STRABISMUS

Marshall M. Parks, M.D.

Attending Staff, Department of Ophthalmology, Children's Hospital;
Attending Staff, Department of Ophthalmology, Washington Hospital Center;
Clinical Professor, Department of Ophthalmology, George Washington University Hospital, Washington, D.C.

Medical Department
Harper & Row, Publishers
Hagerstown, Maryland
New York, Evanston, San Francisco, London

Contents

Preface

The physiology and pathology of ocular motility present a challenge for both the student and practitioner of ophthalmology. The physiology includes not only the myology, but the vastly more complicated neuroanatomy and neurophysiology involved in the motor and sensory aspects of uniocular and binocular macular and extramacular vision. The physiology is further complicated by the overlay of a reflex control system that develops only during infancy and young childhood, linking this area of ophthalmology intimately with pediatric neurophysiology. These major characteristics make comprehension of normal ocular motility difficult, but there are also comparable factors that account for the difficulty in comprehension of the clinical aspects of the multiple aberrations occurring within the ocular motility system. The magnitude of the spectrum of ocular motility disorders and their confusing similar clinical presentations, plus the fact that the majority begin either during infancy or childhood when sophisticated clinical testing is least successful, makes mastering clinical investigation and consistent quality treatment of the ophthalmologic disorder a hardship.

Much of the basic physiology and pathology of ocular motility is a science. However, the clinical management of its disorders remains principally an art. Today's student and practitioner of ophthalmology have inherited a legacy of a myriad of concepts and methods for investigating and treating patients with strabismus and nystagmus. Many of these ideas are worthless, a few are superb and remarkably innovative, but the value of most is mixed—offering something good along with something bad. For an author embarking on the venture of writing a strabismus text the problem created by this legacy must be met. Where to begin, what to include, and how to end the text are not easy questions. This issue was solved here by not reviewing the past—instead I relate the story of strabismus and its therapy as I know and practice it today.

Authorship of this text evolved as an outgrowth of teaching the art of strabismus investigation and management. Participation in the Lancaster Course for the past several years required that the subject of normal ocular motility be presented prior to the clinical subject of strabismus. A teaching manual was essential for the presentation of these lectures. OCULAR MOTILITY AND STRABISMUS is the synthesis of the Lancaster Course and after three revisions appears here as a presentation of my concepts and methods for investigating, evaluating, and treating strabismus.

Although the concepts and techniques of some other authors are discussed in order to present a perspective on some controversial issues, no attempt is made to review in detail all such issues. This would lead to an extensive historical review creating a confusing mass of information for the reader and would not accomplish the aim of the book—the presentation of a succinct text that student and practitioner alike can purchase easily, read swiftly in its entirety, and return to whenever necessary to refresh his memory quickly about any subject discussed in the text. Almost every student and practitioner of ophthalmology needs a plan, a mold, or a model to shape his thinking on strabismus.

Strabismus is a high volume disorder. It is the unusual ophthalmologist who does not find himself actually involved in its management. Even more unusual is the ophthalmologist who is not aggressively seeking a "better way" to manage strabismus disorders. Since perfection in this field is not yet about to overtake us, I hope this book will succeed in supplying the reader with the "better" way he is seeking.

Actually, the reader of this text must realize that little of the material presented is new and exclusively original with the author. I wish to acknowledge the many generations of ophthalmologists who built this rich heritage of ocular motility knowledge. A whole parade of great personages shaped my thinking, many known by name only, but there are a few special people who profoundly and directly affected my ocular motility thinking: Costenbader, Adler, and Burian are among these. Acknowledgment must be given to an equally strong force that continues to shape my thinking—the many residents and fellows who have come under my influence. They, like the strabismus patients themselves, persistently offer inspiration and humiliation, purpose and reward, fulfillment and disappointment. I am especially grateful to William W. Mears, M.D. for his assistance in proofreading the manuscript, to J. Dennis Catalano, M.D. for his photographic assistance, and to my secretaries, Mrs. Marie Anselmo who did the editorial work and Miss Doris Schlaermann who did the typing.

Ocular
Motility
and
Strabismus

1

Extraocular Muscles

Of the body's sense organs, the eye is unique in its capability for independent movement. This feature affords three obvious advantages: (1) a greater field of vision, (2) foveal vision for a large portion of the visual field, and (3) binocular vision for both distance and near.

ANATOMIC FEATURES

LANDMARKS

Several anatomic landmarks on the globe serve as reference points which are important to ocular motility.

The center of rotation is the fixed point within the globe around which all other global points move. The anterior pole is approximately the center of the cornea; the posterior pole is approximately the center of the macula. An axis about which the eye moves extends between the anterior and posterior poles through the center of rotation. This antero-posterior axis is referred to as the Y axis of Fick. An equatorial plane (Listing's plane), lying at right angles to either pole and passing through the center of rotation, divides the globe into anterior and posterior halves. The vertical axis in Listing's plane is the Z axis of Fick, and the horizontal axis is the X axis of Fick. Between these two principal axes, Listing's plane is comprised of an infinite number of oblique axes about which oblique (combined vertical and horizontal) eye movements occur (Fig 1-1).

The direction of rotation about the Y axis of Fick is either toward or away from the midline of the face. More specifically, the 12-o'clock point on the limbus, known as the superior pole of the cornea, is described as rotating medially or temporally about the Y axis.

ARTICULATION

Fundamental to the motility of the eye is its articulation in the orbit. The manner in which muscles are connected between the eye and the orbit and the relationship of their surrounding fascia determine the mechanical features that both produce and limit the motility of the globe.

The eye is suspended within the orbit by a balance of forces. The four rectus muscles exert a significant pull to maintain the eye back against a fat pad which is molded as an intraorbital cushion, while the two oblique muscles exert force to displace the eye forward. Each muscle is encased in its own sheath. The muscles, their sheaths, and the fascial expansions between the muscles (intermuscular septum) form a muscle cone with its apex at the annulus of Zinn and its base occupied by the posterior half of the eye (Fig 1-2). Stuffed into the muscle cone posterior to the eye is a cushion of fat molded to the posterior surface of the eye. Coursing through the fat within the muscle cone are the optic nerve, ophthalmic artery and vein, branches of the oculomotor nerve, and the ciliary ganglion.

Tenon's Capsule

A second fascial structure encircling the posterior two thirds of the eye is Tenon's capsule, extending from the limbus of the cornea to the optic nerve; it is penetrated posterior to the equator of the eye by the four rectus muscles and more anteriorly by the reflected tendon of the superior oblique and the inferior oblique muscle (Fig 1-2). Within the muscle cone, Tenon's capsule constitutes the fascial barrier between the fat cushion of the muscle cone and the sclera. A true space exists between Tenon's capsule and the sclera around the entire spherical surface of the sclera, with attachments of Tenon's capsule to the limbus and the optic nerve. After penetrating Tenon's capsule, the capsules of the four rectus muscles again become joined by the intermuscular septum just as they were in the posterior part of the orbit (Fig 1-3). Anterior to the penetration of the rectus muscles, Tenon's capsule covers the rectus muscles and the intermuscular septum as a cowl. Tenon's capsule is thick, opaque, elastic, and relatively vascular. The intermuscular septum is thin, transparent, elastic, and avascular. Check ligaments (fan-like elastic connections) extend between the muscle capsules and Tenon's capsule. Anterior to the penetration of the rectus muscles into Tenon's capsule, the capsule

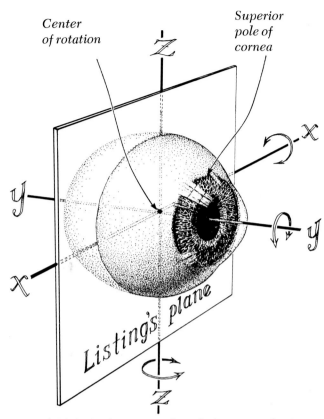

Fig 1-1. Listing's plane passes through the center of rotation of the eye, contains X and Z axes of Fick, and is penetrated by Y axis of Fick.

finally the intermuscular septum. The external fat cushion compartment will not be entered as long as the incision is within 10 mm of the limbus.

Careful and proper surgery on all the extraocular muscles can be performed only if the surgeon is cognizant of all these anatomic facts. The surgeon must make the incision down to the sclera, avoiding penetration of both the extraocular muscle capsule and Tenon's capsule more than 9 mm peripheral to the limbus. Incising the muscle capsule causes profuse bleeding, resulting in hematomas and a blood-filled operative field. Incising Tenon's capsule beyond the area 9 mm peripheral to the limbus penetrates into the orbital fat compartment (Fig 1-3), with extrusion of the fat into the operative field. The mixture of the extruded fat and blood results in fibrofatty proliferation that forms into scarred masses of tissue which distort the normal anatomy, cause cosmetic defects, and restrict the normal motility of the eye. To recess or advance the rectus muscles, the intermuscular septum and check ligaments must be incised. Both the intermuscular septum and the check ligaments should be incised from the insertion of the tendon posteriorly along the peripheral border of the muscle capsule and over the external surface of the muscle capsule for approximately 10 mm. Lastly, the surgeon should avoid placing the incisions of the conjunctiva and Tenon's capsule over the muscle capsule since all three tissues scar together as one unit that is tightly adherent to the scleral surface. This adhesion of all four tissues makes repeat surgery on the muscle difficult and unpredictable; also, this adhesion over the horizontal recti is a cosmetic blemish on the surface of the eye. One can avoid these undesirable features by either placing the incision at the limbus or displacing it away from above the external muscle surface, such as near the inferior or superior conjunctival fornix.

The capsules of the reflected tendon of the superior oblique muscle and the inferior oblique muscle have special anatomic relationships with Tenon's capsule and the intermuscular septum; the surgeon must be aware of these relationships before embarking on surgery to alter the pulling power of these structures. After leaving the trochlea, the superior oblique tendon travels within Tenon's capsule for approximately 8 mm, crosses the space between Tenon's capsule and the intermuscular septum as it approximates the superior rectus muscle, proceeds under the superior rectus muscle, and fans out to a broad insertion 8 to 10 mm farther posteriorly and temporally around the dorsal surface of the sclera. The tendon is within

forms the internal surface of the compartment containing the fat cushion which is external to the muscle cone. The external fat cushion comes forward over the rectus muscles to within 4 mm of their insertions (Fig 1-2). The fat is contained under pressure within both the muscle cone and the extramuscular compartment, and rupture or incision of Tenon's capsule that contains either fat pad allows the orbital fat to protrude forward, often migrating to the external surface of the muscle capsules and creating an unsightly, humped, yellowish mass under the transparent conjunctiva. The conjunctiva is loosely attached by areolar tissue to Tenon's capsule. The intermuscular septum and the areolar tissue extending forward toward the limbus beyond the muscle insertions fuses with Tenon's capsule within 2 mm of the periphery of the limbus. However, peripheral to this fusion of the two fascial layers, the surgeon can cut through three layers before reaching the sclera: first the conjunctiva, second the tissue of Tenon's capsule, and

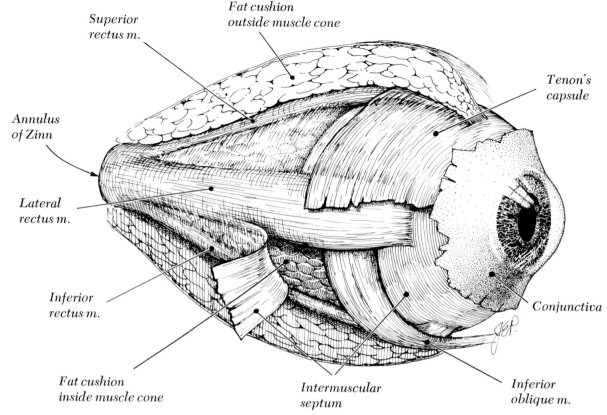

Superior
rectus m.

Fat cushion
outside muscle cone

Tenon's
capsule

Annulus
of Zinn

Lateral
rectus m.

Inferior
rectus m.

Conjunctiva

Fat cushion
inside muscle cone

Intermuscular
septum

Inferior
oblique m.

Fig 1-2. Muscle cone. The muscle cone contains a fat cushion and is surrounded by another. The rectus muscles and intermuscular septums separate the two fat cushions. Tenon's capsule anterior to the penetration of the rectus muscles and intermuscular septums is the inner surface of the compartment containing the fat cushion outside the muscle cone. Tenon's capsule posterior to the penetration of the rectus muscles and intermuscular septums is the anterior surface of the compartment containing the fat cushion inside the muscle cone. Between the lateral margin of the inferior rectus muscle and inferior margin of the lateral rectus muscle the posterior border of the inferior oblique muscle is attached to posterior Tenon's capsule and the anterior border is attached to the intermuscular septum. The inferior oblique muscle capsule is attached by areolar tissue to the capsules of the lateral rectus and inferior rectus muscles.

a delicate sheath which, once it leaves Tenon's capsule and continues on its course to insertion, establishes the same relationship to the intermuscular septum that exists between the capsule of the rectus muscles and the intermuscular septum.

The surgeon should isolate the tendon only after directly visualizing it by elevating Tenon's capsule on a Desmarres lid retractor and pulling the eye downward by a muscle hook under the superior rectus muscle. After dividing the check ligaments between the external surface of the superior rectus muscle and after incising the intermuscular septum along the medial border of this muscle for approximately 9 mm back from the insertion, the glistening white 2-mm superior oblique tendon is visualized as it dips down from the elevated Tenon's capsule to the taut, maximally stretched superior rectus muscle. There the tendon can be plucked out with a small muscle hook, as it now is attached posteriorly only to the intermuscular septum, from which it can easily be separated. The inner face of the elevated, reflected Tenon's capsule along the course of the superior oblique tendon need not and should not be incised, since at this posterior level it is the

inner face of the compartment containing the orbital fat pad which is external to the muscle cone. The bulbar conjunctiva and Tenon's capsule are incised near the superior medial fornix within 9 mm of the limbus, which is anterior to the orbital fat compartment.

Whatever the surgical procedure on the tendon, eg, tenotomy, tenectomy, tuck, or recession, it

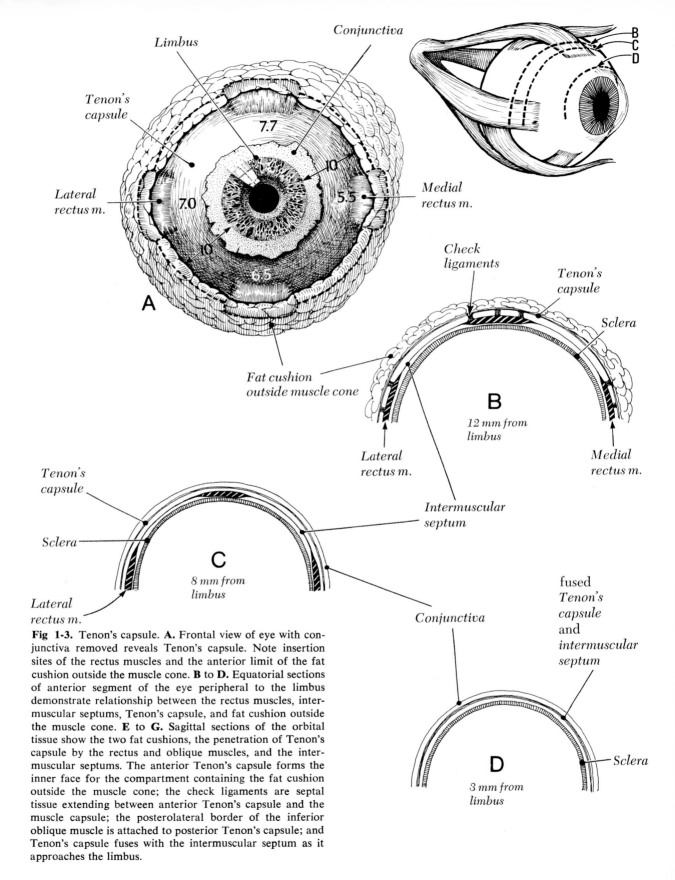

Fig 1-3. Tenon's capsule. **A.** Frontal view of eye with conjunctiva removed reveals Tenon's capsule. Note insertion sites of the rectus muscles and the anterior limit of the fat cushion outside the muscle cone. **B to D.** Equatorial sections of anterior segment of the eye peripheral to the limbus demonstrate relationship between the rectus muscles, intermuscular septums, Tenon's capsule, and fat cushion outside the muscle cone. **E to G.** Sagittal sections of the orbital tissue show the two fat cushions, the penetration of Tenon's capsule by the rectus and oblique muscles, and the intermuscular septums. The anterior Tenon's capsule forms the inner face for the compartment containing the fat cushion outside the muscle cone; the check ligaments are septal tissue extending between anterior Tenon's capsule and the muscle capsule; the posterolateral border of the inferior oblique muscle is attached to posterior Tenon's capsule; and Tenon's capsule fuses with the intermuscular septum as it approaches the limbus.

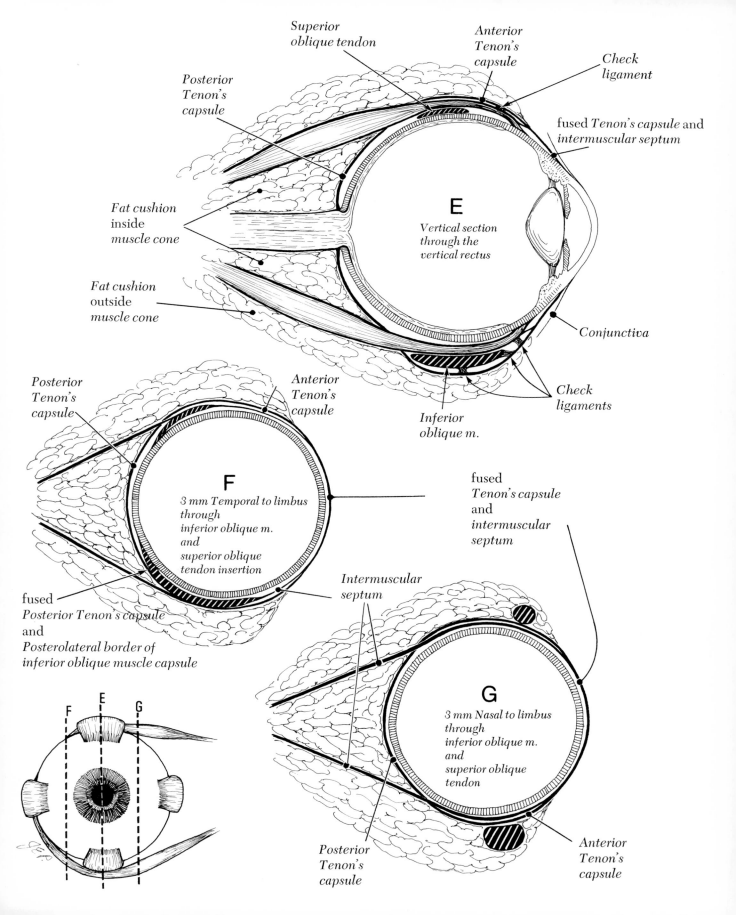

Superior
oblique tendon

Anterior
Tenon's
capsule

Check
ligament

Posterior
Tenon's
capsule

fused *Tenon's capsule* and
intermuscular septum

Fat cushion
inside
muscle cone

E

*Vertical section
through the
vertical rectus*

Fat cushion
outside
muscle cone

Conjunctiva

Inferior
oblique m.

Check
ligaments

Posterior
Tenon's
capsule

Anterior
Tenon's
capsule

fused
Tenon's capsule
and
*intermuscular
septum*

F

*3 mm Temporal to limbus
through
inferior oblique m.
and
superior oblique
tendon insertion*

fused
Posterior Tenon's capsule
and
*Posterolateral border of
inferior oblique muscle capsule*

Intermuscular
septum

G

*3 mm Nasal to limbus
through
inferior oblique m.
and
superior oblique
tendon*

Posterior
Tenon's
capsule

Anterior
Tenon's
capsule

should be performed between the medial border of the superior rectus muscle and the tendon's insertion if possible, thus avoiding the inevitable fibrofatty proliferation and scarring in the superior nasal quadrant that follows tearing and traumatizing Tenon's capsule and extruding the orbital fat from its normal compartment. A tuck or recession procedure requires severance of the tenuous connections between the capsules on the undersurface of the superior rectus muscle and the external surface of the tendon.

The inferior oblique muscle travels for a very short distance from its origin before penetrating Tenon's capsule and proceeds diagonally to cross the external surface of the inferior rectus muscle capsule; it may be rather firmly attached to the inferior rectus muscle capsule, forming Lockwood's ligament. The degree of capsular attachment between these two muscles varies significantly from patient to patient. As the inferior oblique muscle leaves the lateral border of the inferior rectus muscle, its posterior and external capsular surfaces are firmly attached to the surface of Tenon's capsule within the muscle cone; this intimate relationship continues to the point of insertion into the sclera while the internal surface of the muscle presents to the sclera and the anterior border of the capsule is attached to the intermuscular septum. Separating the inferior oblique from Tenon's capsule between the inferior rectus muscle and the insertion requires extremely careful dissection if neither the muscle capsule nor Tenon's capsule are to be punctured. Profuse bleeding occurs with penetration of the muscle capsule, and prolapse of fat from within the muscle cone is associated with penetration of Tenon's capsule. At the insertion of the inferior oblique muscle, the anterior expansions of fascia from the capsule unite it to the scleral surface of the lateral rectus muscle capsule, and posterior expansions of fascia from the inferior oblique muscle capsule fuse with the capsule surrounding the optic nerve. The attachments of the capsule must be severed from the capsules of the lateral rectus muscle and the optic nerve and from Tenon's capsule and the intermuscular septum during recession or resection and advancement of the inferior oblique muscle.

GROSS ANATOMY AND FUNCTION

Medial Rectus Muscle

The medial rectus muscle originates in the orbital apex and courses forward for 40 mm along the medial aspect of the globe; after penetrating Tenon's capsule approximately 12 mm from its insertion, the last 5 mm contacts the eye as it arcs to its insertion 5.5 mm medial to the limbus. The terminal tendinous portion of the muscle is only 4 mm long, so resection of this portion of the muscle results in muscle fibers, rather than tendon fibers, being reattached to the sclera. Furthermore, since muscle tissue is more vascular than tendon tissue, the resection procedure on this muscle is usually associated with considerable bleeding. Recession of the medial rectus muscle is accomplished by retroplacing the tendinous end, thus lessening the inclination to hemorrhage.

Innervation to the medial rectus muscle is by the third cranial nerve, and adduction is produced when the muscle contracts. Adduction is not reduced significantly by recessing the insertion 5 mm. The wraparound section of the terminal 5 mm as it arcs in contact with the globe is simply unwrapped to the quantity of recession desired. This is a tight muscle, and a maximum of 6 mm of resection is possible without also producing resistence to abduction and slight retraction of the eye into the orbit, ie, enophthalmos, and a reduction of the vertical dimension of the palpebral fissure.

Lateral Rectus Muscle

The lateral rectus muscle originates in the orbital apex and courses forward for 40 mm along the lateral aspect of the globe; after penetrating Tenon's capsule approximately 15 mm from its insertion, the last 7 to 8 mm of the muscle contacts the eye as it arcs to its insertion 6.5 mm temporal to the limbus. The terminal tendinous portion of the muscle is 9 mm long, allowing resection to be associated with less bleeding than an equivalent resection of the medial rectus muscle with its short tendon.

Innervation to the lateral rectus muscle is by the sixth cranial nerve, and abduction is produced when the muscle contracts. Abduction is not reduced significantly by recessing the insertion to the equator, a distance of 7 to 8 mm. The wraparound section of the terminal 7 to 8 mm as it arcs in contact with the globe is simply unwrapped to the quantity of the recession desired. This is not a tight muscle like the medial rectus, so excessive resection is less inclined to result in retraction of the eye into the orbit. However, resection of more than 8 mm does offer clinically detectable resistance to adduction.

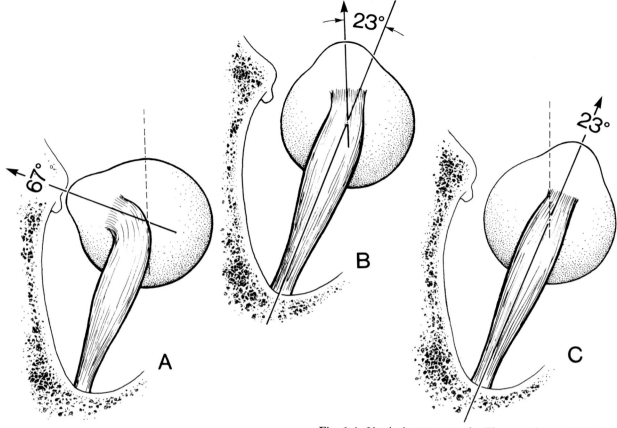

Fig 1-4. Vertical rectus muscle. The superior and inferior rectus muscles course at an angle of 23° with the medial wall of the orbit, giving them vertical action principally in abduction **(C)** and torsional action in adduction **(A)**. In the primary position **(B)** the main thrust of the pulling power is medial to the center of rotation, causing slight adduction action in addition to the cyclovertical action.

Superior Rectus Muscle

The superior rectus muscle originates in the orbital apex and courses forward for 42 mm along the dorsal aspect of the globe, and after penetrating Tenon's capsule approximately 15 mm from its insertion, the last few millimeters of the muscle contact the eye as it arcs to its insertion 7.5 mm superior to the limbus. The terminal tendinous portion of the muscle is 6 mm long.

Innervation to the superior rectus muscle is by the third cranial nerve, and various combinations of vertical, rotary, and horizontal movements of the eye are produced when the muscle contracts. Since the muscle courses forward from the orbital apex at an angle of 23° temporal to the medial wall of the orbit and inserts anterior to the center of rotation of the globe, the movement of the eye produced by the contraction of the muscle varies according to its horizontal starting position (Fig 1-4). Starting from a position of 23° of abduction, the only movement is elevation. Starting from a position of 67° of adduction, the only movement is

intortion. Starting from the primary position, the movement is combined elevation and intorsion plus slight adduction. The adduction results from the midline of the muscle being medial to the center of rotation of the globe when the eye is in the primary position.

Like the medial rectus muscle, the superior rectus muscle is also a tight muscle. Four millimeters is the maximal recession and resection that can be performed without significantly weakening the elevating capacity, producing a resistance to depression, or resulting in retraction of the eye into the orbit. The level of the lower eyelid in reference to the inferior limbus is easily disturbed by excessive surgery on this muscle.

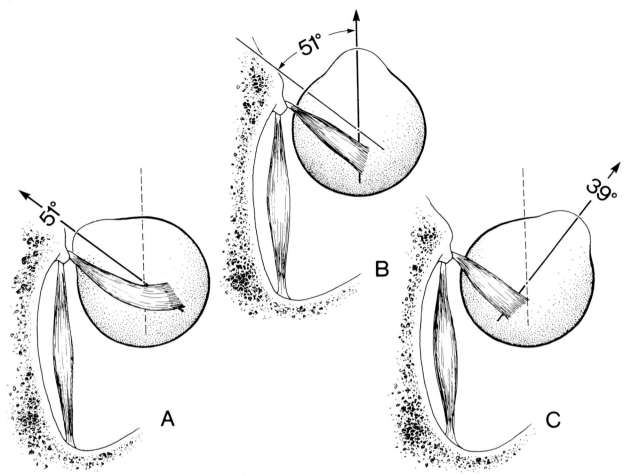

Fig 1-5. Superior oblique muscle. The reflected tendon of the superior oblique muscle and the inferior oblique muscle course on an angle of 51° with the medial wall of the orbit, giving them a cyclovertical action in the primary position **(B)** that becomes principally torsional in abduction **(C)** and vertical in adduction **(A)**. Slight abduction action is also produced, because the pulling power is exerted along a line posterior to the center of rotation.

Inferior Rectus Muscle

The inferior rectus muscle originates in the orbital apex and courses forward for 42 mm along the ventral aspect of the globe; after penetrating Tenon's capsule approximately 15 mm from its insertion, the last few millimeters of the muscle contact the eye as it arcs to its insertion 6.5 mm inferior to the limbus. The terminal tendinous portion of the muscle is 6 mm long.

Innervation to the inferior rectus muscle is by the third cranial nerve, and various combinations of vertical, rotary, and horizontal movements are produced when the muscle contracts. Since the muscle courses forward from the orbital apex at an angle of 23° temporal to the medial wall of the orbit and inserts anterior to the center of rotation of the globe, the movement of the eye produced by the contraction of the muscle varies according to its horizontal starting position (Fig 1-4). Starting from a position of 23° of abduction, the only movement is depression. Starting from a position of 67° of adduction, the only movement is extortion. Starting from the primary position, the movement is combined depression and extorsion plus slight adduction. The adduction results from the midline of the muscle being medial to the center of rotation of the globe when the eye is in the primary position.

Like the medial and superior rectus muscles, the

inferior rectus muscle is also a tight muscle. Four millimeters is the maximal recession and resection that can be performed without significantly weakening the depressing capacity, producing a resistance to elevation, or resulting in retraction of the eye into the orbit. The level of the lower eyelid in reference to the inferior limbus is easily disturbed by excessive surgery on this muscle.

Superior Oblique Muscle

The superior oblique muscle originates in the orbital apex and courses forward for 40 mm along the superior medial wall of the orbit to the trochlea, where it becomes tendinous. After passing through the trochlea, the tendon reflects back temporally, traveling at an angle of 51° with the medial wall of the orbit, and passes dorsally over the globe ventral to the superior rectus muscle and inserts on the sclera's temporal posterior surface. The reflected tendon is 20 mm long and is encased in a sheath. The tendon remains cordlike between the trochlea and the medial border of the superior rectus where its expansion begins.

Innervation to the superior oblique muscle is by the fourth cranial nerve, and various combinations of vertical, rotary, and horizontal movements of the eye are produced when the muscle contracts. Since the reflected tendon delivers the direction of pulling power to the scleral surface when the muscle contracts, the movement of the eye varies according to its horizontal starting position (Fig 1-5). Starting from a position of 39° of abduction, the only movement is intorsion. Starting from a position of 51° of adduction, the only movement is depression. Starting from the primary position, the movement is combined intorsion and depression plus slight abduction; the abduction results from the tendon being posterior to the rotation center of the globe when the eye is in the primary position.

Unlike the tendons of the other muscles, the superior oblique tendon does not lend itself well to recession or resection. Tenotomy or tenectomy and tucking of the tendon are the usual weakening and strengthening procedures performed on the tendon. Tenotomy or tenectomy is performed medial to the superior rectus on the cord portion of the reflected tendon; the tucking procedure is performed temporal to the superior rectus on the expanded portion of the tendon. Tenotomy or tenectomy of the cord portion of the tendon does not completely eliminate the function of the superior oblique muscle. Tucking of the tendon results in a relative inability to elevate the globe in adduction; even a 5- to 10-mm tuck temporal to the superior rectus embarrasses the elevation. Larger tucks, however, create more of an elevation deficit, and tucks medial to the superior rectus result in more embarrassment of elevation than temporally placed tucks.

Inferior Oblique Muscle

The inferior oblique muscle originates on the anterior nasal orbital floor, courses backward and temporally at a 51° angle with the nasal orbital wall, is joined by its sheath to the ventral surface of the inferior rectus muscle, forming Lockwood's ligament, and arcs laterally and posteriorly around the globe to insert into the sclera under the lateral rectus over the macular area. The total length is 37 mm, and there is no obvious tendinous portion.

Innervation to the inferior oblique muscle is by the third cranial nerve, and various combinations of vertical, rotary, and horizontal movements of the eye are produced when the muscle contracts. The movement of the eye varies according to its horizontal starting position. Thus, starting from a position of 39° of adduction, the only movement is extorsion. Starting from a position of 51° of adduction, the only movement is elevation. Starting from the primary position, the movement is combined extorsion and elevation plus slight abduction; abduction results from the muscle being posterior to the center of rotation of the globe when the eye is in the primary position.

Weakening of the inferior oblique muscle is accomplished by recession, myotomy, or myectomy between the temporal border of the inferior rectus muscle and the insertion or between the nasal border of the inferior rectus muscle and the origin. Usually the recession is 10 mm, but it can range from 5 to 15 mm. Myectomy on either side of the inferior rectus is usually 5 mm. The strengthening procedure is usually a combination of resection and advancement of the new insertion, resecting 8 mm and advancing 5 to 6 mm superior to the original insertion. Surgery on the insertion of the inferior oblique demands loosening of the sheath connections between the inferior margin of the lateral rectus muscle and the external surface of the inferior oblique muscle.

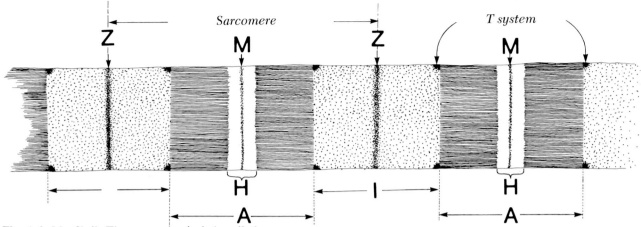

Fig 1-6. Myofibril. The sarcomere includes all the myofibril tissue between Z bands which bisect the light-staining I bands. The M band is a dark, thin line bisecting a clear H band in the center of the dark-staining A band. The T system at the corners of the I band is the conduit for electrical stimulation.

MICROSCOPIC ANATOMY

The extraocular muscles are comprised of skeletal muscle fibers and are separated by connective tissue called the epimysium. Each fiber has a sheath, the sarcolemma. The fiber unit contains the contractile tissue called the myofibrils, the nucleus, and the ground substance called sarcoplasm which contains the fiber's organelles. Cross striations of the myofibrils are created by alternate light- and dark-staining zones, called I and A bands, respectively; to polarized light, the I band is not birefringent, ie, it is isotropic, whereas the A band is birefringent, ie, it is anisotropic. The I band is bisected by a dark line called the Z band. The A band is bisected by a narrow light zone, the H band, and has a dark center line called the M band. The Z band is more prominent than the M band. A contractile unit within the myofibril includes a light and dark zone which is measured from one Z band to the next and is called a sarcomere. Each sarcomere has a tubular arrangement, called the T system, which acts as a conduit for electrical stimulation. Figure 1-6 illustrates the histologic characteristics of the myofibril. When stimulated, the sarcomere contracts by the I and A bands coming together with a ratchet action.

The histologic structure of the extraocular muscles differs from that of the other skeletal muscles. Essentially, the difference is in the unique two-fiber system comprising the extraocular muscles. The fibers of the two-fiber system are histologically different. Resembling the usual skeletal muscles fiber is the fibrillenstruktur fiber, which contains small, well-organized myofibrils surrounded by abundant sarcoplasm, large concentrations of mitochondria, and a nucleus which is usually peripheral. Each sarcomere has an orderly T system. The unique skeletal muscle fiber found in the extraocular muscles is the felderstruktur fiber, containing large, partially fused myofibrils embedded in scant sarcoplasm, a virtual absence of concentrations of mitochondria, and a nucleus which is usually located centrally. These sarcomeres are either devoid of or have a most rudimentary T system. Electron microscopy of the fibrillenstruktur and felderstrukture fibers (Fig 1-7) reveals their histologic differences. Light microscopy of a transverse section of a muscle shows the fibrillenstruktur fibers staining palely with regularly spaced myofibrils, while the felderstruktur fibers stain more densely with irregularly clumped myofibrils.

The fibrillenstruktur fiber is innervated by thick, myelinated nerves that attach by one or two typical motor end-plates. At the synapses, junctional folds of the end-plate are obvious, and within the terminal axon there are many synaptic vesicles. The felderstruktur fiber is innervated by thin, myelinated nerves that have several grapelike nerve terminals extending up and down the full length of the fiber. Only rudimentary junctional folds are seen at the synapse of the nerve terminals and fibers, and the terminal axon contains both granular and agranular synaptic vesicles.

The ratio of nerve fibers to muscle fibers is much greater for the extraocular muscles than for the other skeletal muscles. For example, there is ap-

Fig 1-7. Electron microscopic view of fibrillenstruktur fibers (*above*) and felderstruktur fibers (*below*).

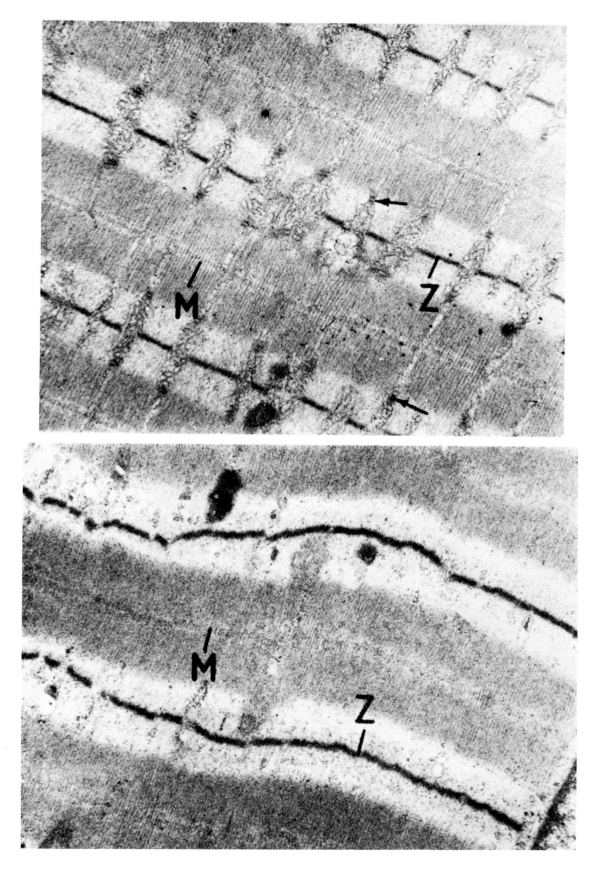

proximately 1 nerve fiber for each 3 extraocular muscle fibers, compared to 1 nerve fiber for each 140 soleus muscle fibers. The 17,000 fibers of the oculomotor nerve supply approximately 40,000 muscle fibers, a ratio of 1:2.7. The ratio of the abducens nerve fibers to muscle fibers is 1:1.8, and the ratio of the trochlear nerve fibers to muscle fibers is 1:1.

PHYSIOLOGIC FEATURES

The fibrillenstruktur fiber corresponds to the striated muscles throughout the body. It contracts rapidly as an ungraded fast twitch in response to a single nerve stimulus; the twitch is accompanied by propagated electrical activity and is followed rapidly by relaxation. The stimulus must be repeated with great frequency to maintain a tetanic contraction. The contraction time of the fibrillenstruktur fiber in the extraocular muscles is exceptionally speedy; for example, in the cat, the contraction time of the medial rectus muscle is 8 msec, that of the gastrocnemius muscle is 40 msec, and that of the soleus muscle is 100 msec.

The felderstruktur fiber contracts slowly and smoothly; the grade of the contraction is proportionate to the repetitive stimuli the fiber receives, and the contraction is maintained before it slowly relaxes. The fiber does not respond to a single stimulus to its nerve. Its contraction is unaccompanied by electrical activity.

The two-fiber system occurs in the skeletal muscles of amphibians, reptiles, and birds, but in mammals it occurs only in the extraocular muscles. The fibrillenstruktur fiber allows the fast optokinetic function so necessary in the saccadic and visual pursuit eye movements. According to Burian (1), the optokinetic function is one of locomotion. The felderstruktur fiber supplies an optostatic function, ie, one of tonicity, that coordinates the positions of the eyes relative to each

other. The optokinetic and optostatic systems function simultaneously.

The extraocular muscles have a rich blood supply similar to that of the cardiac muscles. This facilitates the oxidation of lactic acid and removal of waste products, thus delaying fatigue. In the fibrillenstruktur, the T system and abundant sarcoplasm are important in the rapid transmission of innervation; the concentration of mitochondria is indicative of the large oxidative requirements of the twitch contractions of the fibrillenstruktur. The paucity of these elements in the felderstruktur suggests the oxidative metabolism is considerably less for the slow, tonically contracting fibers.

PHARMACOLOGIC FEATURES

The extraocular muscles are the only skeletal muscles in higher vertebrates that contract under the influence of acetylocholine. The slow, tonic fibers are responsible for this feature, which simulates smooth muscle. In this respect, extraocular muscles behave like the embryonic muscles of mammals, denervated mammalian muscles, and the skeletal muscles of birds and cold-blooded animals.

Succinylcholine causes a response within the extraocular muscles that apparently can be explained only by the presence of a two-fiber system. Initially, succinylcholine and other depolarizing agents cause an increase in base-line tension without disturbing the twitch response. Increasing the dose of succinylcholine is accompanied by graded rises in the base-line tension, but eventually the twitch response is abolished.

REFERENCE

1. Burian HM: Structure and function of the extraocular muscles. In Symposium on Strabismus: Transactions of the New Orleans Academy of Ophthalmology. St. Louis: Mosby, 1971, p 1

2

Eye Movements and Positions

An eye may be moved or displaced in the orbit without rotating about its center of rotation. Such a change in eye position unaccompanied by movement about its center of rotation is a translatory movement. The translatory movement may be in the equatorial plane with the eye being displaced horizontally, vertically, or obliquely; the movement may also occur in the sagittal (anteroposterior) axis, viz, exophthalmos or proptosis and enophthalmos. Translatory eye movements are passive and may be produced by the examiner displacing the eye while palpating the orbital region. Both an expanding lesion in the orbit or a defect in the orbital bones may cause translatory eye movements.

DUCTION

The term "duction" refers to the movement of one eye. A prefix is attached to this word to indicate the direction in which the eye is moved. Duction is accomplished by simultaneous and equally graded contraction and relaxation of antagonistic muscles, in accord with Sherrington's law of reciprocal innervation. Figure 2-1 shows all possible ductions of the right eye, indicating only the contracting muscles.

Abduction is a horizontal movement directed laterally from the vertical axis. It is accomplished by contraction of the lateral rectus muscle and

relaxation of the medial rectus muscle.

Adduction is a horizontal movement directed medially from the vertical axis. It is accomplished by contraction of the medial rectus muscle and relaxation of the lateral rectus muscle.

Supraduction (*sursumduction*) is a vertical movement (elevation) directed superiorly from the horizontal axis of the eye. Supraduction results from the combined contraction of the superior rectus and inferior oblique muscles and the combined relaxation of the inferior rectus and superior oblique muscles. However, as the eye moves into an abducted position the superior rectus becomes the prime elevator muscle; as it moves into adduction the inferior oblique is the principal elevator muscle.

Infraduction (*deorsumduction*) is a vertical movement (depression) inferiorly directed from the horizontal axis. It is the result of the combined contraction of the inferior rectus and superior oblique muscles. However, as the eye moves into an abducted position the inferior rectus becomes the prime depressor muscle; in adduction the superior oblique is the principal depressor muscle.

Combined horizontal and vertical duction moves the eye about an oblique axis in Listing's plane by simultaneous contraction of the elevators or depressors in combination with the medial or lateral rectus muscle and with relaxation of the antagonists of the contracting muscles.

Incycloduction (*intorsion*) is a torsional movement of the eye about the anteroposterior axis so the superior pole of the cornea is displaced medially. Intorsion results from combined contraction of the superior oblique and superior rectus muscles with relaxation of the inferior oblique and inferior rectus muscles. However, as the eye moves into an abducted position the superior oblique muscle becomes the prime intortor, and in adduction the superior rectus muscle is the principal intortor.

Excycloduction (*extorsion*) is a torsional movement of the eye about the anteroposterior axis that displaces the superior pole of the cornea laterally. Extorsion is the result of the combined contraction of the inferior oblique and inferior rectus muscles with relaxation of the superior oblique and superior rectus muscles. However, as the eye moves into an abducted position the inferior oblique muscle becomes the prime extortor, and in adduction the inferior rectus muscle is the principal extortor.

Jampel (1, 2) does not agree with the foregoing classic teaching regarding the vertical and torsional movements of the eyes. He has challenged the concept of oblique muscle action. Based on mathematical considerations, studies of models of the

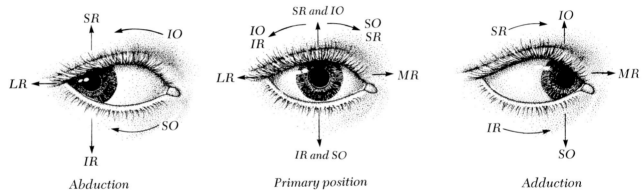

Abduction   Primary position   Adduction

Fig 2-1. Ductions. The horizontal ductions (adduction and abduction) are produced by contractions of the medial rectus (MR) and lateral rectus (LR) muscles. The vertical ductions and cycloductions result from combined contractions of the vertical rectus and oblique muscles. Combined contraction of the superior rectus (SR) and inferior oblique (IO) muscles produce supraduction; combined contractions of the inferior rectus (IR) and superior oblique (SO) muscles produce infraduction. Incycloduction is caused by combined SO and SR contractions, and excycloduction is caused by combined IO and IR contractions. In abduction the vertical rectus muscles are the prime vertical movers and the obliques are the prime torsional movers; in adduction this is reversed.

eye, experimental studies on monkeys, and limited clinical observations, he proposes the following: (1) Elevation and depression, even in adduction, are mainly a function of the superior and inferior rectus muscles. (2) The torsional component of the oblique muscles is the same throughout the range of horizontal eye movement. (3) The abducting component of the oblique muscles does not decrease on adduction but actually increases.

VERSION

"Version" refers to simultaneous movement of both eyes in the same direction; a prefix indicates the direction of the conjugate movement. The muscles in each eye that are the prime movers undergo equally graded contractions in accord with Hering's law of innervation, and for each contracting muscle there is an opposite and equally graded antagonist (Sherrington's law). Figure 2-2 shows the complete range of versions, indicating only the contracting muscles.

Horizontal versions are *dextroversion* and *levoversion*. Dextroversion is accomplished by contraction of the right lateral rectus and left medial rectus muscles and relaxation of the right medial rectus and left lateral rectus muscles. Levoversion is accomplished by contraction of the left lateral

rectus and right medial rectus muscles and relaxation of the left medial rectus and right lateral rectus muscles.

Vertical versions are supraversion (sursumversion) and infraversion (deorsumversion). Supraversion is accomplished by bilateral contraction of the elevator muscles, ie, the superior rectus and inferior oblique muscles, with simultaneous relaxation of the depressor muscles, ie, the inferior recti and the superior obliques. As the eyes move into dextroversion, the right superior rectus and left inferior oblique muscles are the prime elevators; in levoversion the left superior rectus and right inferior oblique muscles are the prime elevators. Infraversion is accomplished by an increase of innervation to the four depressor muscles with an equal decrease of innervation to the four elevator muscles. In dextroversion the prime depressors are the right inferior rectus and left superior oblique muscles; in levoversion the left inferior rectus and right superior oblique muscles are the prime depressors.

Cycloversion is the simultaneous and equal tilting of the corneal superior poles either to the right or the left, ie, either *dextrocycloversion* or *levocycloversion*. Dextrocycloversion is accomplished by contraction of the extortors of the right eye, ie, the inferior rectus and the inferior oblique, and of the intortors of the left eye, ie, the superior rectus and superior oblique, and by relaxation of the intortors of the right eye, ie, the superior rectus and superior oblique muscles, and of the extortors of the left eye, ie, the inferior rectus and inferior oblique muscles. In dextroversion the most effective dextrocycloverters are the right inferior oblique and left superior rectus muscles. In levoversion the most effective dextrocycloverters are the left superior oblique and right inferior rectus muscles. Levocycloversion is accomplished by an increase of innervation to the extortors of the left eye and the intortors of the right eye with a simultaneous de-

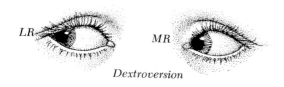

Dextroversion

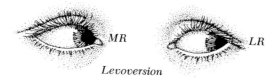

Levoversion

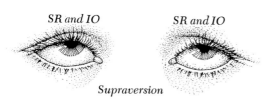

Supraversion

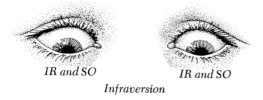

Infraversion

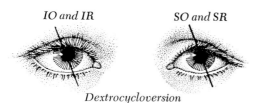

Dextrocycloversion

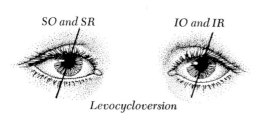

Levocycloversion

crease of innervation to the intortors of the left eye and the extortors of the right eye. In dextroversion the primary levocycloverters are the left inferior rectus and right superior oblique muscles; in levoversion the left inferior oblique and right superior rectus muscles are the prime levocycloverters.

VERGENCE

Vergence is the simultaneous and equal movement of the eyes in opposite directions; a prefix attached to "vergence" indicates the direction of the disjugate movement. The muscles that are the prime movers undergo equally graded contractions in accord with Hering's law of innervation, and for each contracting muscle there is an opposite and equally graded relaxing antagonist (Sherrington's law). Figure 2-3 shows all possible vergence movements, indicating only the contracting muscles.

Horizontal vergences are *convergence* and *divergence*. Convergence is accomplished by contraction of the medial rectus muscles and relaxation of the lateral rectus muscles. Divergence is accomplished by contraction of the lateral rectus muscles and relaxation of the medial rectus muscles.

Vertical vergences are designated as *positive* and *negative*. Positive vertical vergence is elevation of the right eye with simultaneous depression of the left; negative vertical vergence is depression of the right eye with simultaneous elevation of the left. Each is accomplished by elevators contracting in one eye and depressors contracting in the other with equal and simultaneous relaxation of their antagonistic muscles.

Cyclovergence is equal and simultaneous tilting of the corneal superior poles either inward or outward, ie, either *incyclovergence* or *excyclovergence*. Incyclovergence is accomplished by simultaneous contraction of all intortors, ie, the superior recti and superior obliques, and relaxation of all extortors, ie, the inferior recti and inferior obliques.

Fig 2-2. Versions. Horizontal versions (dextroversion and levoversion) are produced by contractions of yoked medial rectus (MR) and lateral rectus (LR) muscles. Vertical versions result from combined contractions: superior rectus (SR) and inferior oblique (IO) muscles causing supraversion and inferior rectus (IR) and superior oblique (SO) muscles causing infraversion. Torsional versions are produced by combined contractions of intortors of one eye (SO and SR) and extortors of the other (IO and IR); dextrocycloversion results from right eye extortors and left eye intortors contracting, and levocycloversion results from right eye intortors and left eye extortors contracting.

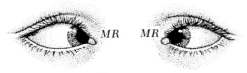

Convergence

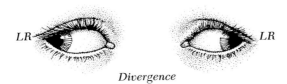

Divergence

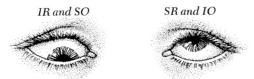

Positive vertical vergence

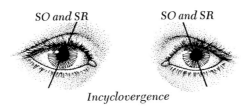

Negative vertical vergence

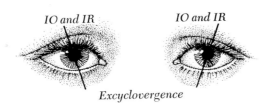

Incyclovergence

Excyclovergence

Excyclovergence is accomplished by an increase of innervation to the extortors and an equal decrease of innervation to the intortors.

EYE POSITION

The *primary position* is the position the eyes assume when fixating an infinitely distant object straight ahead. Because of the difficulty in meeting the requirement that the fixation point be at an infinite distance and because of the little practical difference in the horizontal alignment of the eyes between fixating at infinity compared with fixating at 6 meters, fixating at 6 meters is considered primary position. The primary position can be maintained with the head erect or with the head tilted to either shoulder. By comparing the eye alignment in the primary position in the various tilted positions of the head, the physician can evaluate the muscles that have a combined torsional and vertical action. Levocycloversion is stimulated with the head tilted to the right; dextrocycloversion is stimulated with the head tilted to the left. A weak cyclovertical muscle produces both a torsional and a vertical deviation that changes as the head is tilted, although the eyes never move out of the primary position.

Secondary positions are any variation of eye position other than primary and include near fixation positions, cardinal positions, and midline vertical positions.

Near fixation position is fixating straight ahead at a point at some arbitrary distance less than 6 meters. Distances for near fixation usually range from 0.25 to 1 meter, with most near testing of the eye alignment performed at 0.33 meter. Comparison of the near fixation and primary position alignments provides information about the reflex involving convergence and accommodation.

Fig 2-3. Vergences. Horizontal vergences are produced by simultaneous contractions of the medial rectus (**MR**) muscles of each eye (convergence) or the lateral rectus (**LR**) muscles of each eye (divergence). The vertical vergences are caused by combined superior rectus (**SR**) and inferior oblique (**IO**) muscle contractions in one eye and inferior rectus (**IR**) and superior oblique (**SO**) muscle contractions in the other; the right eye elevators and the left eye depressors simultaneously contract to produce positive vertical vergence, and the right eye depressors and the left eye elevators simultaneously contract to produce negative vertical vergence. The torsional vergences result from simultaneous combined contractions of either the two intortors (**SO** and **SR**) of both eyes, producing incyclovergence, or the two extortors (**IO** and **IR**) of both eyes, producing excyclovergence.

Patient's right   *Patient's left*

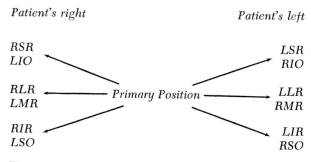

Fig 2-4. Primary position and cardinal positions. The pulling power of each of the six extraocular muscles compared to its yoke is assessed by studying the movements of the eyes from the primary position into the cardinal positions. Illustration is arranged as if the patient is facing the examiner. RSR, right superior rectus; LIO, left inferior oblique; RLR, right lateral rectus; LMR, left medial rectus; RIR, right inferior rectus; LSO, left superior oblique; LSR, left superior rectus; RIO, right inferior oblique; LLR, left lateral rectus; RMR, right medial rectus; LIR, left inferior rectus; RSO, right superior oblique.

Cardinal positions are the six gaze positions that compare the horizontal and vertical eye alignments produced by the six extraocular muscles. One muscle of each eye is the prime mover to achieve the six positions. Figure 2-4 illustrates the primary position and the six cardinal positions; it also indicates the prime movers of each eye (yoke muscles) that achieve these positions. Three of the cardinal positions are in dextroversion; the other three are in levoversion. In each levoversion and dextroversion, elevation and depression are compared in addition to straight right and straight left gaze.

Midline positions are straight up and down from the primary position. They are of value in comparing the elevating and depressing capabilities of each eye, but they do not allow a discreet comparison of isolated muscles of each eye, as the cardinal positions do. This is because each eye has two elevator and two depressor muscles, and both effectively move the eye in a vertical plane away from the primary position. The midline position is all-important for assessing horizontal alignment change as the eyes move in the vertical plane; this change consists of the A and V patterns.

Eye position relative to the position of the upper lid is of interest. Normally, the upper lid follows the vertical eye movements, the eye maintaining approximately the same relative position to the superior limbus during movement. However, during sleep the levator muscle becomes atonic, permitting the lid to cover the eye; the eyes are usually elevated and diverged (Bell's phenomenon), and this movement is simulated by forced closure of the eyelids. Prying the eyelids apart as the patient attempts to forcibly close them reveals the eyes to be markedly elevated.

REFERENCES

1. Jampel RS: The action of the superior oblique muscle. Arch Ophthalmol 75:535, 1966
2. Jampel RS: The fundamental principle of the action of the oblique ocular muscles. Am J Opthalmol 69:623, 1970

3

Innervation
of
the
Extraocular
Muscles

Cranial nerves III, IV, and VI course forward together in the lateral portion of the cavernous sinus, entering the orbit through the superior orbital fissure (Fig 3-1).

Cranial nerves III and VI enter the orbit within the muscle cone. Cranial nerve III divides into a superior and an inferior branch. Some fibers of the superior branch terminate directly in the superior rectus muscle; others traverse this muscle and end in the levator muscle. The inferior branch first sends fibers to the medial rectus and inferior rectus muscles, then passes beneath the optic nerve to the floor of the orbit between the lateral rectus and inferior rectus muscles, and ends in the inferior oblique muscle. Cranial nerve VI proceeds directly to the mesial surface of the lateral rectus muscle.

Cranial nerve IV enters the orbit through the superior orbital fissure lateral and superior to the annulus of Zinn. It courses superiorly and radially as it proceeds forward in close proximity to the periorbita of the orbital roof, crossing over the levator muscle to enter the superior oblique muscle.

OCULOMOTOR

The nucleus of cranial nerve III is a complex of both paired and midline motor cells located in the mesencephalon at the cross-sectional level of the superior colliculus in the midline just ventral to the central gray substance. It is a mass of paired cells, 5 mm long, positioned rostrocaudally. The paired masses are angled toward one another so that on dorsoventrad cross section the nucleus appears as a V with the apex pointing ventrally. Motor cells that send fibers to the respective muscles innervated by cranial nerve III are arranged in the arms of the V in a rostrocaudal and dorsoventrad direction.

For almost a century the relationship of these cells has caused controversy between neuroanatomist and neurophysiologist. Studies have provided conflicting results depending on whether a retrograde degeneration technique or a Horsley-Clarke stereotaxic electrode technique with minimal excitatory currents was used. Results have also varied according to whether the study was performed on rodents, cats, or monkeys. Currently the accepted study is that of Warwick (1) (1953 to 1956) (Fig 3-2), performed on monkeys with retrograde degeneration techniques. The nuclear motor cells of the various fibers innervating the extraocular muscles supplied by cranial nerve III are arranged rostrocaudally in the arm of the V like a group of overlapping bananas. The dorsal nucleus sends uncrossed fibers to the ipsilateral inferior rectus muscle, the intermediate nucleus to the ipsilateral inferior oblique muscle, and the ventral nucleus to the ipsilateral medial rectus muscle. The paramedian nucleus sends fibers which decussate to the contralateral superior rectus muscle. The central caudal nucleus sends fibers to innervate both levator muscles. There is an anterior median nucleus (Edinger-Westphal), composed of small, multipolar cells, which sends uncrossed parasympathetic fibers into the oculomotor nerve. Caudally it is a paired nucleus; rostrally the paired cell masses fuse into a median mass. However, there is no evidence that the fibers emanating from this fused mass have any representation other than homolateral. An inconstant single median mass of large stellate cells, Perlia's nucleus, is found about the middle third of the oculomotor complex. Since phylogenetically it is more prevalent in species having frontal eyes and high-grade binocularity, it was once speculated that this nucleus might be a convergence center. However, retrograde degeneration experiments indicate that fibers from this nucleus innervate intraocular muscles in the same manner as the Edinger-Westphal nucleus.

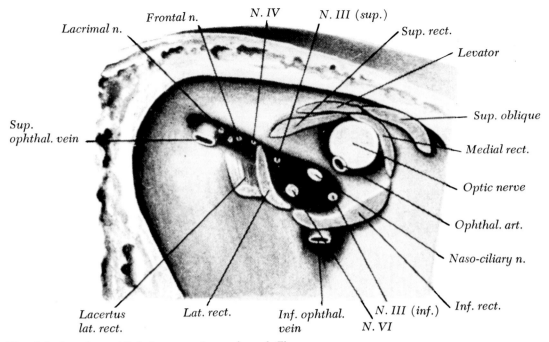

Fig 3-1. Superior orbital fissure and annulus of Zinn. Cranial nerves III and VI enter orbit within the muscle cone, but cranial nerve IV enters lateral to annulus of Zinn.

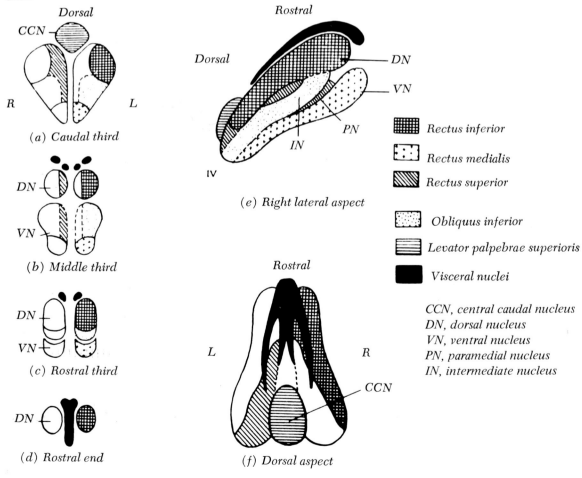

(a) Caudal third

(b) Middle third

(c) Rostral third

(d) Rostral end

(e) Right lateral aspect

(f) Dorsal aspect

- Rectus inferior
- Rectus medialis
- Rectus superior
- Obliquus inferior
- Levator palpebrae superioris
- Visceral nuclei

CCN, central caudal nucleus
DN, dorsal nucleus
VN, ventral nucleus
PN, paramedial nucleus
IN, intermediate nucleus

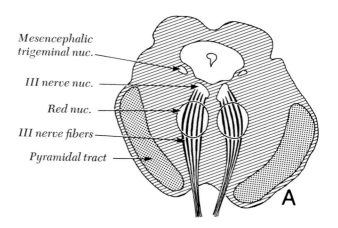

Mesencephalic
trigeminal nuc.

III nerve nuc.

Red nuc.

III nerve fibers

Pyramidal tract

A

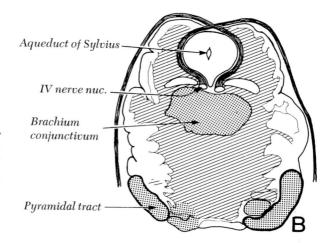

Aqueduct of Sylvius

IV nerve nuc.

Brachium
conjunctivum

Pyramidal tract

B

◀ **Fig 3-2.** Warwick's arrangement of the cranial nerve III nuclei, illustrating the pattern of motor cells in the brainstem that send fibers to each of the ocular muscles innervated by this nerve.

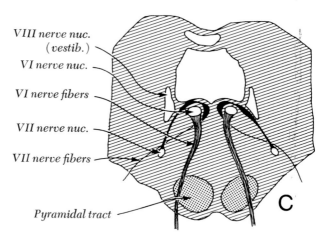

VIII nerve nuc.
(vestib.)

VI nerve nuc.

VI nerve fibers

VII nerve nuc.

VII nerve fibers

Pyramidal tract

C

Fig 3-3. Cross sections of the brainstem. **A.** Through superior colliculus, showing cranial nerve III nuclei with intramedullary fibers. **B.** Through inferior colliculus, showing cranial nerve IV nuclei with intramedullary and extramedullary fibers. **C.** Through floor of fourth ventricle, showing cranial nerve VI nuclei with intramedullary fibers.

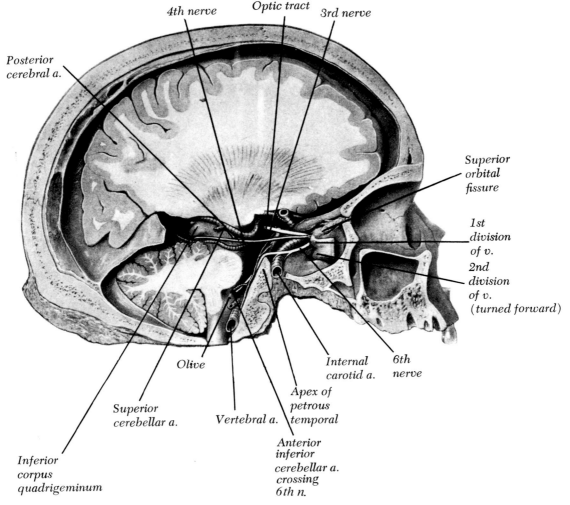

4th nerve

Optic tract

3rd nerve

Posterior
cerebral a.

Superior
orbital
fissure

1st
division
of v.
2nd
division
of v.
(turned forward)

Olive

Internal
carotid a.

6th
nerve

Superior
cerebellar a.

Vertebral a.

Apex of
petrous
temporal

Inferior
corpus
quadrigeminum

Anterior
inferior
cerebellar a.
crossing
6th n.

Fig 3-4. Extramedullary course of cranial nerves III, IV, and VI.

The intramedullary fibers of cranial nerve III course ventrally through the red nucleus and the substantia nigra and emerge from the brainstem in the interpeduncular fossa at the rostral margin of the pons (Fig 3-3, *A*). There are no decussations.

The extramedullary fibers course forward through the subarachnoid space to penetrate the dura mater at the posterior clinoid process, entering the cavernous sinus (Fig 3-4).

TROCHLEAR

The nucleus of cranial nerve IV is a paired group of motor cells located in the mesencephalon at the cross-sectional level of the inferior colliculus in the same relative position as the nucleus of the third nerve, appearing as caudal extensions of this nucleus.

The intramedullary fibers course dorsally, curving around the central gray substance and decussating as they emerge from the roof of the midbrain (Fig 3-3, *B*).

The extramedullary fibers course ventrally and rostrally as they wrap themselves around the brainstem. They travel through the subarachnoid space and proceed to the level of the posterior clinoid process, penetrating the dura mater to enter the cavernous sinus (Fig 3-4).

ABDUCENS

The nucleus of cranial nerve VI is a paired group of motor cells located in the pons in the floor of the fourth ventricle near the midline, just medial and at the rostral end of vestibular nuclei and proximal to the center for lateral conjugate gaze (Fig 3-3, C). The medial longitudinal fasciculus lies just medial to the nucleus of the sixth nerve.

The intramedullary fibers course ventrally through the tegmentum of the pons without decussation to emerge on the ventral surface of the brainstem at the caudal border of the pons on either side of the midline.

The extramedullary fibers course forward and laterally over the petrous tip of the temporal bone and under the petrosphenoid ligament. (This space is called Dorello's canal.) They then pierce the dura mater to enter the cavernous sinus where they lie in contact with the wall of the carotid artery (Fig 3-4).

REFERENCE

1. Warwick R: Representation of the extraocular muscles in the oculomotor nuclei of the monkey. J Comp Neurol 98:449, 1953

4

Supranuclear Centers and Pathways of Eye Movements

Supranuclear innervation results in movements of the eyes in certain directions rather than a contraction of any individual muscle. Supranuclear innervations produce either conjugate or disjugate eye movements.

BRAINSTEM SUPRANUCEAR CENTERS AND PATHWAYS

Brainstem supranuclear centers and pathways serve both conjugate and disjugate gaze. Although relatively little is difinitely known about these centers and pathways, some facts important to ocular motility have been proven. For example, sectioning the brainstem caudal to the inferior colliculi does not interfere with vertical movement of the eyes but does eliminate horizontal conjugate movement. The brainstem supranuclear centers for lateral conjugate gaze (parabducens nuclei) are just lateral to the nucleus of the sixth nerve and are either part of or immediately proximal to the vestibular nuclei. Some fibers from the center for lateral conjugate gaze connect directly with the homo-

lateral nucleus of the sixth nerve; others bypass the sixth nerve and join the contralateral medial longitudinal fasciculus to ascend the brainstem and reach the contralateral nucleus of the third nerve (Fig 4-1). Presumably they have synapsed with the motor cells within the nucleus of the third nerve that supply fibers to the ipsilateral medial rectus. This arrangement permits the lateral rectus of one eye and the medial rectus of the other to contract and move both eyes in the same horizontal direction.

The corticopontine fibers mediating horizontal gaze (Fig 4-1) arrive at the center for lateral conjugate gaze after leaving the corticofugal pathways; they then decussate at the level of the nucleus of the third nerve while descending in the periaqueductal gray matter. This causes an impulse arising in the right cortex to reach the left center for lateral conjugate gaze, evoking a simultaneous movement of both eyes to the left.

The brainstem supranuclear centers for vertical conjugate gaze are located rostrally in the mesencephalon. They are at the level of the nucleus of the third nerve (superior colliculi) within the central gray matter of the pretectal zone and posterior commissure. They are probably in the midline where there are separate centers for upward and downward gaze. Fibers are sent directly to the nuclei of the third and fourth nerves. The corticofugal fibers to the supranuclear centers for vertical conjugate gaze probably travel through the internal capsule and in the cerebral peduncle with those for horizontal conjugate gaze, parting company with the latter as they decussate at the level of the nucleus of the third nerve. Fibers ascend from the caudal area of the brainstem (Fig 4-1), probably via the medial longitudinal fasciculus, connecting the vestibular nuclei to the centers for vertical conjugate gaze. These probably convey the labyrinthine reflex, auditory reflex, tonic neck reflex, and cerebellar influence as they pertain to vertical gaze.

The brainstem supranuclear design subserving torsional conjugate movements is probably intimately interrelated with or else actually the same as the vertical supranuclear pattern, since all muscles that move the eyes vertically also move them torsionally. Hence, they are referred to as cyclovertical muscles.

Serving disjugate gaze, the supranuclear center for convergence is in close proximity to the centers for vertical conjugate gaze; this is supported by ample experimental and clinical evidence. Therefore, the supranuclear center for convergence is probably in the midline central gray matter of the mesencephalon at the level of the nucleus of the third nerve. The connections of the corticofugal and

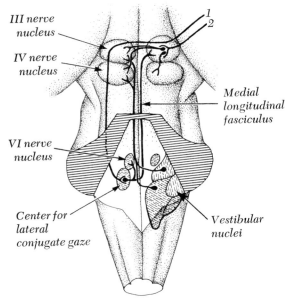

III nerve nucleus

IV nerve nucleus

Medial longitudinal fasciculus

VI nerve nucleus

Center for lateral conjugate gaze

Vestibular nuclei

Fig 4-1. Brainstem, showing supranuclear and internuclear pathways for conjugate and disjugate gaze.

medial longitudinal fasciculi are probably similar to those serving vertical conjugate gaze. Nothing is known about the centers and pathways for divergence or those serving vertical and torsional disjugate movements.

CEREBRAL SUPRANUCLEAR CENTERS AND PATHWAYS

Two areas of the cortex are identified as controlling oculogyria: one is located in the frontal lobe, the other in the occipital lobe. Actually, oculogyric activity has been shown to be represented extensively over the cerebral surface: eye movements have been induced by stimulation over as much as one third of the hemispheric surface. Experiments in unanesthetized animals with electrodes implanted in the central cortex demonstrate this. Anesthesia depresses cerebral activity so that all but the foci in the frontal and occipital lobes are rendered inexcitable.

The frontal lobe mechanism controls voluntary eye movement, while the occipital lobe involuntarily moves the eyes in response to visual stimuli; the latter are called optomotor reflexes. The voluntary eye movements are rapid and jerky and are called saccadic movements (up to 400°/sec); the involuntary movements are slow and smooth (8° to 25°/sec). Both the voluntary and optomotor cortical mechanisms produce conjugate and disconjugate eye movements.

VOLUNTARY CORTICAL CENTERS AND PATHWAYS

The cortical centers for voluntary movement are located in area 8 (Brodmann's areas), which is at the posterior end of the second frontal convolution. Fibers descend through the basal ganglia with or without synapses, passing through the anterior arm of the internal capsule near the knee, in apposition to the fibers traveling from the facial muscles (Fig 4-2). This intimate relationship is responsible for the oculogyric crisis associated with disease of the basal ganglia. The fibers continue in the pyramidal tracts until departing in the mesencephalon at the area of the superior colliculus to decussate and proceed to the brainstem supranuclear centers.

Conjugate Gaze

Stimulating the right Brodmann area 8 causes levoverted eyes since the right cortex is connected by the corticopontine fibers to the left center for lateral conjugate gaze. Sudden loss of one oculogyric center of the frontal lobe results in a transient inability to deviate the eyes to the opposite side on command, but following movements of the optomotor pathway persist. Removing the tone of one cortical center allows the other to act unopposed. Within a few weeks after destruction of one side, the remaining cortical center assumes the task of carrying out voluntary lateral gaze in both directions. The frontal centers for eye movements and for head movements are in close apposition, which explains why voluntary eye movements are so commonly associated with identical head movements.

Vertical movements are produced only by (1) simultaneously stimulating both right and left Brodmann's area 8 with equipotential electrodes, (2) severing the horizontal recti before stimulating either the right or the left frontal cortex, (3) destruction of the centers for lateral conjugate gaze, and (4) total transverse sectioning of the brainstem caudal to the mesencephalon. Usually stimulating the upper part of Brodmann's area 8 depresses the eyes, and stimulation of the lower part of Brodmann's area 8 elevates the eyes.

Apparently there is no voluntary ability to move the eyes torsionally. Anyone can move his eyes horizontally or vertically on command, but he cannot move them into dextrocycloversion or levocycloversion.

Disjugate Gaze

There is a brisk convergence response of the eyes to command which is associated with accommodation and pupillary constriction. Therefore, the true

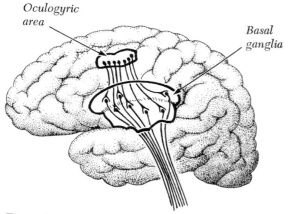

Fig 4-2. Frontal lobe oculogyral pathways, illustrating synapse of the fibers in the basal ganglia.

response is more than voluntary convergence, ie, it is the voluntary application of the synkinetic near reflex. Some erratic convergence responses have been produced by excitatory experimental techniques.

There is no voluntary divergence counterpart to convergence. Also, there are no vertical or torsional disjugate movements initiated by the voluntary cortical center.

CORTICAL CENTERS AND PATHWAYS FOR INVOLUNTARY MOVEMENTS

The centers are located in Brodmann's areas 17, 18, and 19 (striate, parastriate, and peristriate areas). Experimentally, the least potential is required for the strongest eye movements when the calcarine fissure (area 17) is stimulated.

The development of following movements of the optomotor system is delayed in infants until after the development of the voluntary movements produced by the frontal oculogyric centers. There are pathways that interconnect the occipital and frontal centers; the frontal centers are dominant. For example, equipotential stimulation of right frontal and left occipital areas results in eye movements to the left. Willed movements interrupt fixation and optomotor movements; otherwise, fixation would be frozen on a certain object.

Efferent fibers descend from the occipital cortex parallel and medial to the optic radiation. They pass through the posterior end of the internal capsule to the superior colliculus (Fig 4-3); some of the fibers decussate to descend to the most rostral portion of the opposite center for lateral conjugate gaze in the pons, and others end in the supranuclear centers serving conjugate and disjugate gaze which are located in the mesencephalon.

Conjugate Gaze

The eyes deviate to the side opposite the side of the occipital lobe which is stimulated. Acute lesions of the occipital lobe produce transient deviation of the eyes to the homolateral side.

The optomotor fibers to the pontine nuclei differ somewhat from the frontal corticopontine fibers in their course. The optomotor fibers apparently do not have synaptic connections with the basal ganglia as do fibers from the frontal lobe, since bilateral lesions of the basal ganglia are associated with loss of voluntary eye movements but not with loss of horizontal optomotor eye movements. Also, destruction of the superior colliculi eliminates optomotor movements but not voluntary movements, indicating some intimate relationship between the optomotor corticopontine fibers and the superior colliculi that is not shared with the fibers from the frontal lobe.

The optomotor reflex enables the corrective duction of the eye to keep a moving image continuously projected on the fovea. The same reflex assures continued proper positioning of the eye so that a static object of regard stays imaged on the fovea; this is called the fixation reflex.

There are optomotor fibers controlling vertical and torsional movements. Although little is known about them, they probably have the same corticofugal pathways from the cortex to the level of the superior colliculi as do the optomotor fibers relaying horizontal movements.

Optokinetic nystagmus is caused by a fixation point moving in a constant direction. There is a slow or following phase, followed by the rapid recovery phase. A lesion in the parietal lobe near the angular gyrus disturbs this jerk-type nystagmus.

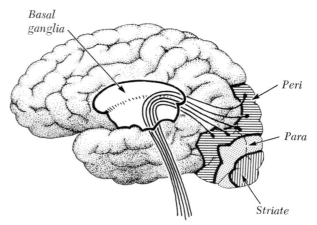

Fig 4-3. Occipital lobe oculogyral pathways, illustrating fibers passing through posterior end of the internal capsule.

The right parietal lobe controls the optokinetic response to the right side (objects moving to the patient's right initiate a slow-phase eye movement to the right, followed by rapid restoration toward the midline); the left parietal lobe controls the homolateral jerk nystagmus response to objects moving to the left. The optic radiations and the optomotor fibers must be in close proximity in the parietal lobe, since lesions in the posterior two thirds of the visual pathways not only cause hemianopsia but also an absence or diminution of optokinetics to a test target moving toward the side of the lesion.

Optokinetic responses may be used to objectively measure visual acuity. By grading the spacing between stripes on a drum rotating at a constant speed, the examiner can determine the smallest separation between stripes which evokes the optokinetic response, thus yielding a measure of the angular acuity. It may be used in testing visual acuity in infants, illiterates, malingerers, and animals.

The slow phase of optokinetic nystagmus depends on optomotor pathway function, while the rapid phase is a function of the voluntary motor pathway of the frontal lobe. A bilateral disease of the frontal lobe or severance of the association pathways between the frontal and occipital lobes results in the eyes responding to the slow phase of the jerk nystagmus without the rapid phase following. This is seen in the clinical condition called oculomotor apraxia, which can be acquired secondary to disease or injury or which can be congenital due to improper embryonic development of the above-described frontal lobe centers or association pathways. Due to lack of control of the frontal lobe, the patient's fixation is "locked" by the oculogyric reflexes of the occipital lobe, since normally the frontal lobe reflexes, being stronger than occipital lobe reflexes, constantly break fixation. A patient with oculomotor apraxia can only break fixation by closing or blinking his eyes, covering his eyes, or turning his head far enough to interrupt visual contact. These patients have normal control over voluntary vertical gaze as evidenced by instantaneous and precise vertical fixation movements and normal vertical optokinetic nystagmus. Reading is a problem for these patients.

Vertical optokinetics have no distinction similar to that of horizontal optokinetics in laterally localized cerebral lesions. However, ablation of the superior colliculi destroys the vertical optokinetic response without disturbing horizontal optokinetics. The first sign of pinealoma, even before Parinaud's signs of defective vertical eye movements and convergence, is reported to be an absence of upward following movements in testing of vertical optokinetics.

Disjugate Gaze

The portion of the optomotor system that deals with disjugate gaze is most important in strabismus, because both the motor aspect of the fusion reflex and the accommodative convergence portion of the synkinetic near reflex are disjugate optomotor reflexes.

The fusion reflex enables a corrective disjugate movement of the eyes to eliminate or diminish disparity of similar images on the right and left retinas. The pathways serving the motor component of this reflex probably descend from the occipital cortex to the level of the superior colliculi in the brainstem. The designs of their distribution from this point to the nuclei of the third, fourth, and sixth nerves are unknown. All three planes of disjugate movements, ie, horizontal, vertical, and torsional fusional vergences, are served by this reflex.

Accommodation is the response to insufficient vergence of light waves striking the macula, resulting in an image that is more sharply focused. The motor response is actually a synkinetic reflex, there being constriction of the pupil and convergence in addition to accommodation. Collectively, this synkinetic response comprises the near reflex. Thus, at some unknown level between the cortex and the brainstem the accommodation reflex is linked to the other two responses. It is not known whether linkage occurs at the cortical level, in a supranuclear center in the brainstem, or in the nucleus of the third nerve. However, Jampel (1) found that in monkeys, stimulating areas 19 and 22 by the faradic method evoked the near reflex.

EXTRACEREBRAL MECHANISMS OF EYE MOVEMENTS

Extracerebral eye movements are those produced by or modified by reflexes other than those provided by the two cerebral pathways and centers. The extracerebral mechanisms use the same brainstem supranuclear system that mediates cerebral eye movements.

LABYRINTHINE REFLEXES

The most important source of reflex tonus for the extraocular muscles, other than visual, is that mediated by the vestibular division of the eighth nerve. This complex mechanism correlates changes in posture with movements of the eyes by means of reflexes which are divided into static reflexes, due to changes in the position of the head with respect to gravity, and statokinetic reflexes, resulting from movement of the head through space, ie, acceleration and deceleration.

Each labyrinth exerts a continuous tonic innervation tending to turn and to rotate the eye to the opposite side, ie, the right labyrinth causes levoversion and levocycloversion, while the left labyrinth produces dextroversion and dextrocycloversion. Removal of one labyrinth, therefore, results in the eyes being turned toward that side, due to the unopposed action of the intact labyrinth. Although the tonus from the labyrinth is constantly present, it may be inhibited by other sources of tonus, eg, by voluntary innervation from the frontal oculogyric centers. Only conjugate movements are produced by labyrinthine reflexes; no disjugate movements are possible.

The otolith apparatus effects a static reflex, repositioning the eyes within the orbits with changes in the position of the head in respect to gravity. The otolith apparatus includes the utriculus and the sacculus, but the function of the sacculus is unknown. The utriculus is a sensory organ having afferent fibers which lie in the vestibular nerve and which synapse with cells in the vestibular nuclei. It is stimulated during changes in the position of the head by otoliths, which are little sandlike concretions contained in the macula. Reflexes arising in these organs cause tonic sustained contractions of the extraocular muscles and other skeletal muscles which may produce changes in the posture of the eyes and the body. The altered tonus is preserved as long as the new position of the head is maintained.

Movements initiated by the otolith apparatus tend to keep the eyes fixed in position, despite a change in the position of the head. It is as though the static reflexes exert an influence on the eye muscles, making them resistant to change in the position of the eyes. The otolith apparatus is not as important in man as in the lower animals, but the following reactions occur. (1) When the head is placed in flexion, the eyes are tonically deviated upward; when the head is held in extension, the eyes are tonically deviated downward. (2) When the head is inclined to either shoulder, the eyes undergo torsion in the opposite direction on the anteroposterior axis in such a way as to compensate for the altered position of the head and thus preserve their original orientation. This compensatory torsional movement is brought about by the increase in tonus of those muscles which tend to keep the vertical meredian of the cornea erect as the head is tilted to the right or left. If the head is tilted to the right, for example, levocycloversion must be produced in both eyes to keep the vertical

meridians vertical. Therefore, there must be an increase in tone in the right superior oblique and right superior rectus muscles and in the left inferior oblique and left inferior rectus muscles. At the same time the tonus of each of the antagonistic muscles is diminished.

The utricular reflex does not send innervation to the medial or lateral recti; it sends innervation only to the cyclovertical muscles. The magnitude of response is one tenth of the total head movement. For every 10° of head tilt, the eyes cyclovert 1° in the opposite direction. The maximal response is produced by approximately 60° of head tilt.

The vestibular system effects a statokinetic reflex, repositioning the eyes within the orbits with acceleration and deceleration of head movements. The vestibular system includes three semicircular canals within that portion of the petrous bone known as the bony labyrinth. Each canal has a bulbous enlargement on one end, called the ampulla, which contains the sensitive crista. The canals contain a fluid, the endolymph, that is displaced when the head is moved. Provided that the movement is carried out with a minimal velocity, pressure rises at one end of the canal and falls at the other end. This results in a change in pressure on the mounds of sensory hair cells imbedded in the cristae. Pressure of the fluid on the cristae creates a chemical reaction which in turn causes a change in the potential in the vestibular fibers of the eighth nerve. Acceleration or deceleration of head movement is the necessary stimulus for exciting the cristae, the minimum being 1° to 3°/sec. Vestibular fibers from the cristae enter the vestibular nuclei; the impulses are transmitted from there to the various nuclei of the oculomotor nerves through the posterior longitudinal bundle.

The semicircular canals constantly send a base level innervation to each of the ocular muscles, but there is no change in the tonus of any set of muscles of the two eyes unless an imbalance between the right and the left vestibular apparatus has occurred. Extirpation or destruction by disease of one labyrinth causes a deviation of both eyes to the side of the destroyed labyrinth. Similarly, stimulation of the semicircular canals on only one side causes the eyes to slowly move away from the stimulated side. The eyes escape the vestibular driving force after moving a few degrees and are whipped back to the primary position (saccadic movement) by the voluntary oculogyric system of the frontal cortex. The recurrence of the slow vestibular movement and the opposite saccadic movement in a rhythmic manner is identified according to the rapid phase; the direction of the slow phase is the vestibulogenic portion of the nystagmus. It is a manifestation of the attempt to maintain the position of the eyes which existed before acceleration or deceleration of the head movement.

The three sets of semicircular canals are so arranged that head movement in the sagittal plane produces a vertical response in eye movement and head movement in the coronal plane produces a torsional (rotary) response in eye movement.

TONIC NECK REFLEX

Whenever the head is turned on the shoulder, the occipitoatlantal and atlantoaxial joints are stretched and send proprioceptive impulses which influence the position of the eyes into the central nervous system. These impulses also reach the oculomotor nuclei through the posterior longitudinal bundle. However, these impulses are not nearly as effective in man as they are in the lower vertebrates.

AUDITORY REFLEX

Practically all of the sense organ systems at one time or another modify the tonus of the ocular muscles. A loud noise causes the eyes to turn reflexly to the side from which the noise seems to come.

PAIN REFLEX

A painful stimulus applied to the side of the face causes the eyes to turn involuntarily to the origin of the pain.

EXTRAPYRAMIDAL SYSTEM

Maintenance of muscle tone and of the rhythm characteristic of normal movements depends on the interfunctioning of the following (Fig 4-4): (1) the prefrontal cortex, (2) the basal ganglia, (3) the three masses in the midbrain, ie, the subthalamic nucleus of Luys, the red nucleus, and the substantia nigra, (4) the bulbotegmental reticular formation, and (5) the cerebellum.

The extrapyramidal system provides accurate, instantaneous, smooth movement of the eyes to obtain a certain position; it also enables the eyes to sustain this exact position for an indefinite time. Without the control of this system, eye movements are inaccurate (overshooting compensated by redress), unsustained (tend to drift back to center position), and jerky (cogwheel-type movements).

PROPRIOCEPTION FROM OCULAR MUSCLES

Cooper et al (2) have recorded afferent impulses from nerve endings on a single fiber of the inferior

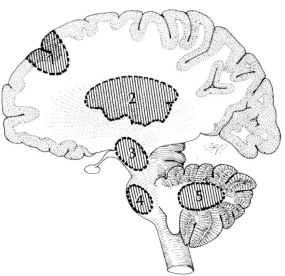

Fig 4-4. Extrapyramidal system, consisting of five interfunctioning masses of motor cells: (1) the prefrontal cortex; (2) the basal ganglia; (3) midbrain cell masses, including the subthalamic nucleus of Luys, the red nucleus, and the substantia nigra; (4) the bulbotegmental reticular formation; and (5) the cerebellum.

oblique muscle and from nerve fibers in the oculomotor nerve. The discharges were increased during relaxation (stretching) of the muscle fiber and decreased on contraction. They also found that these same discharges on muscle stretching occur in fibers of the fourth and sixth cranial nerves. In the ocular muscles of goats, impulses in response to stretching have been recorded in a mass of cells considered to be part of the nucleus of the fifth nerve.

Breinin (3) has electromyographically demonstrated a base level of firing in the medial and lateral rectus muscles while the eye is in the primary position. The firing diminishes when the muscles are severed from the globe. Stretching the muscle increases the firing to the base level found in the primary position, but the firing can never be increased beyond this level, no matter how great the tension applied to the muscle. Normally, on right and left gaze there is simultaneous, exact augmentation and decrease of firing in agonist and antagonist. This is lost when the medial and lateral rectus muscles are disinserted from the globe before right and left gaze are attempted. When abduction is attempted, a sudden violent burst of firing occurs in the lateral rectus; this abruptly ceases when adduction is tried next. This is followed by a sudden, violent burst of medial rectus firing, but this occurs only after there is an interval during which neither muscle fires. Therefore, disinsertion releases the tension normally experienced by attached antagonistic muscles; this accounts for the loss of the finely graded augmentation and decrease which characterizes Sherrington's law of reciprocity for opposite-acting muscle groups.

This basic stretch reflex of the extraocular muscles is probably the substitute for proprioception. Such a feedback mechanism permits constantly accurate adjustments to be made in optomotor responses to visual stimuli. This is extremely important in monocular fixation in which constant corrections have to be made to ensure continued projection of the image onto the fovea. The eye is never still while fixating, and these ever-present little quivering moverments are called micronystagmus or physiologic nystagmus.

Man is devoid of a sense of ocular position. If his vision is cut off, the subject is unaware of any passive eye movement. Furthermore, when asked to move his eyes while one eye is occluded and immobilized with forceps, the patient believes the covered, unmoving eye has made the same large angle of movement as the uncovered, unrestrained eye. This lack of sense of ocular position can also be demonstrated with afterimages: the afterimage is perceived as moving although the eye movement was prevented by restraint. Futhermore, a person with extraocular muscle palsy has the impression that the eye has moved according to the degree it was willed to move, when actually no movement has occurred; there is no sense of ocular position to inform him otherwise.

REFERENCES

1. Jampel RS: Representation of the near-response on the cerebral cortex of the Macaque. Am J Ophthalmol 48(2):573, 1959

2. Cooper S, Daniel P, Whitteridge D: Muscle spindles and other sensory endings in the extrinsic eye muscles: The physiology and anatomy of these receptors and their connection with the brainstem. Brain 78:564, 1955

3. Breinin GM: Electromyographic evidence for ocular muscle proprioception in man. Arch Ophthalmol 57:176, 1957

5

Single Binocular Vision

While vision in itself is a complex phenomenon, single binocular vision is even more complex. There are three requisites for vision: (1) light stimulus, (2) sensation, and (3) perception. The light stimulus for vision is the visible spectrum of electromagnetic waves. Adequate light creates a sensation in the retinas which is transmitted to the cortex. Interpretation of the light sensation is the perception process. This chain reaction of light—sensation—perception is vision; lack of any of the three results in no vision.

THE LIGHT STIMULUS AND THE RESPONSES

MONOCULAR VISION

Four separate characteristics of the light stimulus are identifiable: frequency and duration, intensity, the length of the light waves, and the angle of the light waves entering the eye.

Frequency and duration of the light stimulus are characteristics that evoke the on-off light sensation, providing the perception of a flickering or sustained light.

Intensity of the light stimulus is the characteristic that creates a light sensation ranging from weak to strong, providing perception of a dim or a bright light. The intensity of the stimulus is graded according to the volume of light waves that enters the eye per unit of surface area.

The length of the light wave is a characteristic that is appreciated only by the cones of the retina and not by the rods. Regardless of the wavelength, the sensation of the rods is unvaried, and they perceive only light. However, the cones in photopic vision respond with a multitude of varied sensations related to the wavelength of the light stimulus, each sensation providing varied color perception.

The angle at which the light enters the eye is the characteristic of the stimulus that determines which retinal neuroepithelial photoreceptor is stimulated. Each stimulated photoreceptor has the innate ability to register the specific angle formed by the light wave and the corneal surface; this is the basis for spatially identifying the direction the light wave was traveling in reference to the eye at the time it entered. Photoreceptors in the fovea register a zero directional value, and the image projected here is perceived as centered in the visual field. A stimulated receptor nasal to the fovea localizes objects in space to the temporal side of center, a superior receptor localizes inferior to center, and so on; the number of degrees that each localization is away from center is equal to the number of degrees the stimulated neuroepithelial element is displaced from the fovea.

Since the refracting surfaces of the eye exert a constant effect on all penetrating light waves, the characteristic of the light wave angle, applied to an infinite number of light waves emanating from a multitude of light sources and comprising a patterned spatial stimulus, is the basis for the contoured image that projects onto the retina. Light waves emanating from objects in the visual field form miniaturized retinal images. The contour of each image is determined by the contrast produced between stimulated and unstimulated photoreceptors. The contrast sensation results in the perception of shape, size, and relative location of objects. Since the fovea possesses the highest resolving power for contrast sensation, projection of images onto this area results in maximal perception of contour, known as "best visual acuity." The fixation point is the spatial location of the object of regard. The fixation line (visual axis) is a line drawn between the fixation point and the fovea (Fig 5-1). The best visual acuity is obtained and maintained for the object of regard by a complex visuomotor reflex designed to steer the fixation line; this is known as the fixation reflex. It is an involuntary reflex mediated through the optomotor pathways, but it may be interrupted by disturbing innervations arriving at the extraocular muscles over the voluntary oculogyric pathways of the frontal lobe, the vestibular pathways, and the auditory and pain pathways.

The development of the fixation reflex is first manifest when the infant is 5 to 6 weeks old. The

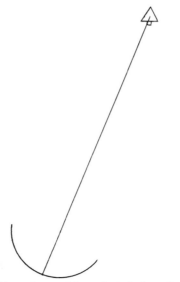

Fig 5-1. Object of regard is projected along the visual line and imaged on the fovea.

eyes follow a light or a bright object for a few degrees, but once fixation is interrupted, reestablishment is slow. At 3 months of age, the infant maintains fixation in all fields of gaze and reestablishes fixation instantly after interruption. By 4 months of age, he begins to associate fixation with grasping movements to attempt to bring the target of fixation to his mouth. Oral identification of the object will continue for the next four months before being replaced by visual and tactile identification. By the time the child is 9 years old, the constant conditioning of the fixation reflex gives it an irreversible quality comparable to an unconditioned reflex; however, below this age, cessation of the conditioning process results in its reversal, as manifest by amblyopia. Total deprivation of stimuli from birth, which thwarts the development of the fixation reflex, results in the reflex never developing unless corrective treatment eliminates the stimulus deprivation during approximately the first six months of life. At least, this has been the clinical experience from treating patients with unilateral congenital cataracts. Partial deprivation of stimuli, as occurs in strabismus and anisometropia, results in a less severe amblyopia and a relatively better prognosis for normal development of the fixation reflex with treatment. Treatment of strabismus amblyopia by 4 years of age is almost always successful, but the favorable prognosis decreases as the age at which treatment is initiated increases.

Absence of the maculas, bilateral congenital destructive disease of the maculas, or bilateral macular images below a critical threshold of intensity and clarity in infants results in a pendular nystagmus first appearing at 3 to 4 months of age. The nystagmus is present only when fixation is attempted, indicating a defect in the steering mechanism of the fixation line. This phenomenon suggests the degree of frustration associated with bilateral thwarted development of the fixation reflex. Nystagmus does not occur in patients with unilateral absence of the fixation reflex, even when their normal eye is occluded.

Best monocular visual acuity demands the combination of three essentials: a maturely developed fixation reflex which is normal in both its sensory and motor aspects, precise stimulation, and maximal attention directed to the object of regard. According to clinical observation, the fixation reflex appears to mature by the time the child is approximately 9 years old, since visual acuity remains in a state of flux until then, decreasing with disuse of the reflex and returning to normal with use. Sensory abnormalities of the reflex may be in the retina or within the visual pathways. Abnormalities in the retina include lack of anatomy, such as absent maculas associated with albinism and aniridia, and deficient cone physiology, such as is found in achromatopsia. A lesion disrupting the macular fibers within the visual pathways is equally detrimental to monocular acuity. Motor abnormalities of the reflex are exemplified by congenital nystagmus. Ptosis, opacities within the optic media, and abnormalities in refraction preclude precise stimulation of the fovea with intense and sharp images. Inattention to the foveal image as occurs in strabismus, however, is the most common cause for submaximal visual acuity.

Strabismus and absence of bifoveal vision (disregard of the image on one fovea) in the immature person accounts for more amblyopia than all other causes combined.

SINGLE BINOCULAR VISION

Fusion of the sensation produced by the light stimulus in each eye into a unified perception is single binocular vision.

Frequency and Duration

Frequency and duration of the light stimulus at normal binocular viewing produces nothing different from monocular viewing. However, in the laboratory, viewing circumstances in which the eyes are alternately stimulated with flickering illumination in opposite cycles (when one light comes on, the other goes off), cycled below the critical flicker-fusion rate, results in binocular perception of a sustained light but monocular perception of flickering light.

Intensity

Intensity of the light stimulus also is appreciated no differently in binocular vision than in monocular except under rare circumstances. Two inadequate light stimuli directed separately into each eye are not additive in the sense that fusing the two can make one adequate stimulus. A dim light is not seen as brighter nor is a bright light further intensified by seeing with two eyes rather than one. In fact, the binocular response is the same as the monocular response unless the light intensity entering each eye is different. In the laboratory this situation can be produced by presenting a black formless surface to one eye and a white formless surface to the other. The fused perception is a lustrous metallic gray, ever changing by darkening and lightening in various portions as a result of retinal rivalry. In the absence of single binocular vision this phenomenon does not occur, and the sustained impression of either a black or a white surface prevails. A similar phenomenon occurs in patients with a unilateral acquired cataract. When viewing a formless, illuminated background, such as the sky, the patient experiences a binocular dimness that clears on closing the cataractous eye and becomes dimmer on closing the normal eye; however, retinal rivalry persists when both eyes are open, manifest by the sky increasing and decreasing in dimness in a patchy manner. This particular phenomenon is called interference.

Wavelength

The length of the light wave under normal binocular viewing circumstances has little opportunity to yield a perception that differs from the monocular perception. However, the wavelength entering each eye may be controlled by laboratory techniques; dissimilar lengths create some binocular perceptions totally different from monocular perception. Different colored lights presented to each eye are perceived either in color fusion, according to the scheme for mixture of colored lights rather than for mixture of pigments, or in color rivalry. Color fusion occurs only when a very few combinations of colors of specific wavelengths are presented to the two eyes (Table 5-1). Otherwise, color rivalry of the two different formless fields of colored illumination occurs, with an everchanging patchy perception of the two. In the absence of single binocular vision, either one or the other persists

TABLE 5-1. Color Fusion

	Stimulus to One Eye	Stimulus to Other Eye	Fused Perception
Complementary colors	red	+ greenish blue	= white
	orange	+ cyan blue	= white
	yellow	+ indigo blue	= grayish white
	greenish yellow	+ violet	= white
Tints	red	+ white	= pink
	orange	+ white	= yellow
	yellow	+ white	= green
	green	+ white	= yellow
	violet	+ white	= salmon pink

as a sustained, colored, formless field. Tints also are appreciated in patients with single binocular vision by presenting white light to one eye and a certain monochromatic light to the other. The diluted fused perception is a tint according to the scheme of mixing colored lights (Table 5-1).

In sensory testing of a patient's binocular mechanism, color rivalry and color fusion (tints) form the basis of some tests. For example, a red lens before one eye and a green lens before the other causes the white viewed light to be perceived in color rivalry if the patient has single binocular vision; otherwise, either a red or a green sustained light is perceived. Another is the red glass test, in which a red glass is held before one eye while the patient views a white light. The patient with binocular vision sees a pink light (diluted from red), whereas the patient without fusion sees either a red or a white light.

Angle

The angle of the light waves entering the eye has a significant response in binocular vision that is lacking in monocular vision. This is attributable to an object in space projecting onto retinal photoreceptors in each eye which have identical localizing values. A pair of such neuroepithelial elements are referred to as corresponding points. The foveas, as well as all other photoreceptors of the two eyes having identical directional values, are corresponding points. Images projected on these points are localized in space with the same values as though the image were on only one of the corresponding points.

Lines drawn from corresponding points through the nodal points of the eyes intersect in space either at a distance remote from the eyes or at a distance close to the eyes, depending on whether the eyes are fixating a distant point or are converged to fixate a near point. An imaginary plane including

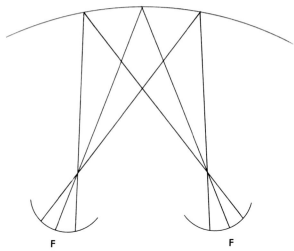

Fig 5-2. A horopter is an infinitely thin plane drawn through all object points that project onto corresponding retinal points.

all the points of intersection of these lines in space is a horopter (Fig 5-2). The horopter is an infinitely thin toric plane in space with its center being the fixation point. The concavity of the distant horopter is almost nil, but it increases with increasing nearness of the fixation point and consequent convergence. An object located at any point on this plane projects images onto corresponding points on the retina. The angle formed by the intersecting fixating axes equals all the other angles formed by lines drawn from all other corresponding retinal points that intersect at the horopter.

FUSION. All objects projecting onto corresponding points have their two images fused into one perception. However, the neurophysiology involved in binocular vision does not impose such a rigid requirement for fusion. Objects projecting onto slightly disparate retinal points also may be fused provided the disparate images are within a critical limit. The quantity of disparity between foveal images which permits fusion is small, but the permissible disparity of images which allows fusion increases progressively for the more peripheral retinal points. Therefore, for each retinal point in an eye there is a definable corresponding area in the retina of the opposite eye within which the same image must project if the two images are to be fused into one (Fig 5-3). The more eccentric the retinal point from the fovea, the larger is the corresponding area in the other eye.

Lines drawn from the boundaries of the corresponding areas through the nodal point of the eye

intersect in space with the line extending from the corresponding point of the opposite eye. The line from the temporal boundary intersects the line of the corresponding point of the opposite eye proximal to the horopter (Fig 5-3). As in the construction of the horopter, if all points of the interesecting lines proximal to the horopter from retinal points and the temporal boundaries of the corresponding retinal areas of the opposite eye were connected by a plane, the proximal boundary of Panum's area would be defined. The distal border is defined by joining together all intersecting points distal to the horopter of lines from retinal points in an eye and the nasal boundaries of the corresponding retinal areas of the opposite eye. Since the peripheral retinal points have corresponding areas with larger dimensions than central retinal points, Panum's area is most narrow at its center and widens as it proceeds peripherally from the fixation areas.

The retinal area in one eye that corresponds to the fovea in the other eye permits inexact alignment of the visual axes. While the object of regard is imaged on the fovea of one eye it is slightly displaced from the fovea in the other, yet single

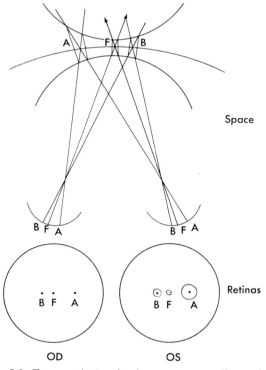

Fig 5-3. Every retinal point has a corresponding retinal area in the opposite eye, upon which the similar image must project to be fused. The more peripheral retinal points have larger corresponding retinal areas.

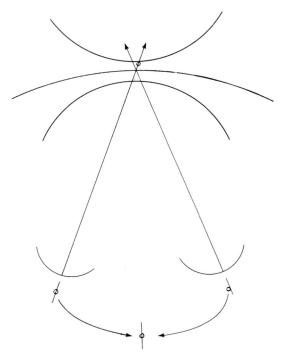

Fig 5-4. Similar foveal images disparate up to 14 minutes of arc are fusible.

binocular vision occurs. The inexact fixation of one eye (Fig 5-4) in the presence of single binocular vision is fixation disparity. It is physiologic, and the maximal quantity of deviation of the fixation axes may range between 10 and 14 minutes of arc. If there is a convergent deviation (esodeviation) of the eyes, although fusion keeps the deviation latent to the degree that single binocular vision is possible (esophoria), there is an esofixation disparity. Divergent deviation (exodeviation) is accompanied by exofixation disparity.

SIMULTANEOUS PERCEPTION. All objects distal or proximal to Panum's area project their images outside corresponding retinal areas and are not fused. An object outside Panum's area projects its images on the retinas with a degree of disparity exceeding the boundary of the retinal area of one eye that directionally corresponds to the retinal point receiving the image in the other eye. Although these disparate images are not fused, if they are perceived simultaneously, the object is simultaneously localized by the eyes to different places in space (diplopia). All object points not located within Panum's area are diplopic unless one is inattentive to these object points. The diplopia due to simulaneously perceiving object points distal and proximal to Panum's area is physiologic, since it is

a component of normal single binocular vision. Diplopically perceived objects proximal to the fixation point project onto nasal retinas (Fig 5-5). Bitemporal disparity and binasal disparity of the retinal image are the basis of binocular parallax, used in differentiating the relative proximal-distal location of object points in reference to the object of regard. Actually, the interretinal distance is a more accurate concept, since object points displaced laterally to the object of regard may evoke physiologic diplopia yet produce neither bitemporal nor binasal disparity. For example, an object point proximal to Panum's area but to the right of the object of regard is imaged on the left half of each retina. Although this cannot be described as bitemporal retinal image disparity, the localizing function of these disparate images is equivalent to this. However, it is more accurate to describe the interretinal image distance (used similarly to interpupillary distance) projected on each retina from the proximal, peripheral, nonfusible object point as exceeding the interretinal distance of the images

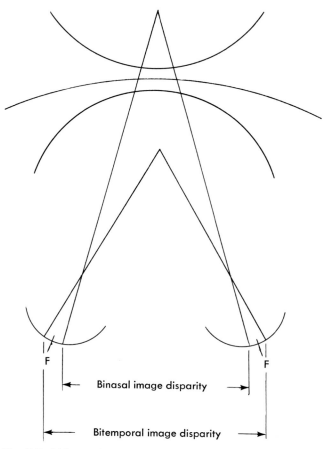

Fig 5-5. Object points proximal or distal to Panum's area produce physiologic diplopia.

projected from the object of regard. Interretinal image distances exceeding the object of regard interretinal image distance localize the object point proximal to the object of regard. The reverse is true for interretinal image distances less than the distance projected by the object of regard (Fig 5-5).

STEREOPSIS. Within Panum's area, another single binocular vision phenomenon, stereopsis, occurs. Stereopsis is the perception of the third dimension (relative nearness and farness of object points within Panum's area) obtained from fusible but disparate retinal images. The same clues are used in stereopsis for determining relative nearness and farness of object points within Panum's area as those used in physiologic diplopia to determine the same feature about object points proximal and distal to Panum's area. The stereopsis determination hence is made on the basis of differences in interretinal distances of the fusible images within Panum's area: the greater interretinal image distances are projected by nearer object points, and the lesser interretinal image distances are projected by further object points.

Fusion, stereopsis, and simultaneous perception are the three essential but distinctly different perceptual phenomena comprising single binocular vision. All three usually are capable of functioning simultaneously, although simultaneous perception is usually suppressed unless voluntarily recognized. There are some congenitally esotropic patients who, after their eyes have been straightened by surgery, only develop the simultaneous perception and fusion

components of single binocular vision and never develop stereopsis. Binocular vision is a cortical function, and there probably are separate specialized cortical cells for each component. The cortical cells serving simultaneous perception, fusion, and stereopsis are conjectured to be completely individualized in their morphology, physiology, and distribution frequency throughout the cortex. They are indeed considered to be three separate neurophysiologic phenomena, sharing only the fact that they function only during the cortical processing of the images projected simultaneously on each retina.

TERMINOLOGY. Unfortunately, at the turn of the century Worth (1) used the term "fusion" for what is now called "single binocular vision." He then introduced the terms "first-, second-, and third-degree fusion. He described first-degree fusion as a simultaneous awareness of dissimilar targets presented in a haploscopic device (Fig 5-6), eg, targets such as a fish to one eye and a bowl to the other (Fig 5-7, *A*). Second-degree fusion was the unifying of similar targets having one minor dissimilarity, presented to each eye in the composite, eg, the target being a flying insect with two sets of wings, half of the wings presented to the right eye and the other half presented to the left eye (Fig 5-7, *B*). Furthermore, the similar portions of each slide incited a motor response allowing fusional vergence amplitudes to be recorded; however, simultaneous awareness of dissimilar images on each retina has no capability of evoking a motor response. Third-degree fusion as described by Worth was the integrating of similar but disparate targets,

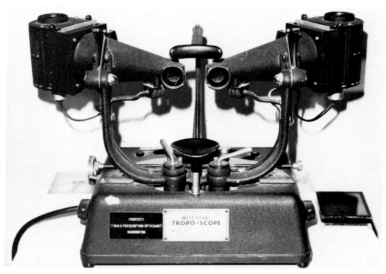

Fig 5-6. Haploscopic instrument (major amblyoscope).

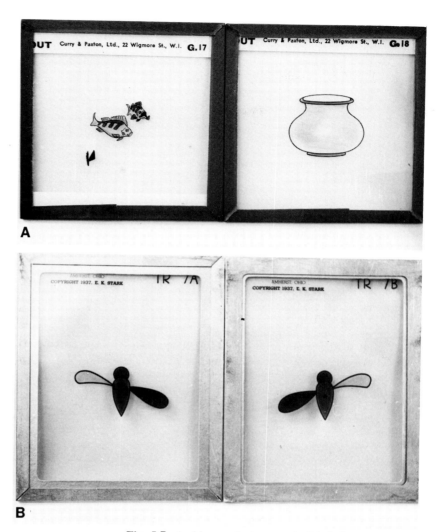

A

B

Fig 5-7. Amblyoscopic targets. **A.** Dissimilar. **B.** Similar.

obtaining a perception of stereopsis, eg, targets of a swing with the frame portion of the swing presented to each eye as nondisparate images but the rope and the swing board suspended from the swing frame presenting either bitemporal or binasal retinal image disparity, making the rope and swing board appear swung toward or away from the swing frame when viewed in the haploscope.

Worth did not imply all three degrees of fusion invariably occurred. Instead, the inference was that fusion may be so rudimentary that only first-degree is present; second-degree fusion was better than only first-degree; but if the patient possessed third-degree fusion, the fusion mechanism was excellent.

Gradually Worth's terminology was altered, and "fusion" was replaced with "single binocular vision." Worth's "first-degree fusion" became known as "simultaneous perception"; "second-degree fusion" was simply altered to "fusion"; and "third-

degree fusion" was changed to "stereopsis." However, many examiners who were indoctrinated with the haploscopic assessment of single binocular vision continue to think and articulate in terms of Worth's three levels of fusion rather than the three perceptual phenomena that characterize single binocular vision.

The difficulties created by Worth's "three levels of fusion" concept start with the first level. The simple explanation of simultaneous perception as the ability to simultaneously perceive dissimilar slides presented to the viewer in a haploscope does not do justice to this complex neurophysiologic component of single binocular vision. Simultaneous perception of dissimilar images in a haploscope is the laboratory equivalent of only one of the two separate visual circumstances occurring in ordinary seeing that demonstrate simultaneous perception.

The dissimilar targets in the haploscope simulate the circumstance that occurs in a nonstrabismic person who sees the visual environment at a distance by one eye and the obstruction precluding the same view by the other eye. Being aware of the distinctly different images simultaneously projecting onto the retinas is only one of the visual circumstances that reveals simultaneous perception. The other visual circumstance occurring during ordinary seeing that demonstrates simultaneous perception is being attentive to an object outside Panum's area. This produces physiologic diplopia, ie, the similar images are not fused because they are too disparate. The haploscopic dissimilar targets used by Worth are unable to produce this visual circumstance attendant with similar disparate images. Thus, Worth's first-degree fusion test does not reveal the important neurophysiologic fact that physiologic diplopia is simultaneous perception outside Panum's area.

Therefore, simultaneous perception occurs in response to two separate visual circumstances: one is the appreciation of dissimilar images (Worth's first-degree fusion), and the other is appreciation of similar images too disparate to fuse (physiologic diplopia). Simultaneous perception merely records the simultaneous spatial localizing values inherent for that moment within the retinal points of the two eyes when such points are presented with nonfusible visual stimuli, regardless of whether the visual stimuli are similar or dissimilar images.

The main difficulty with Worth's concept of fusion and stereopsis is that his terminology of second- and third-degree fusion does not impart the fact that fusion and stereopsis are separate perceptual responses to different visual stimuli arising only from within Panum's area. Although stereopsis is different from fusion, which the newer terminology suggests, both occur simultaneously in normal single binocular vision. In fact, simultaneous perception, fusion, and stereopsis all occur simultaneously as three distinct phenomena comprising single binocular vision; they are not a system of grading the quality of single binocular vision, as Worth implied.

Since fusion and stereopsis both occur in response to visual stimuli arising from within Panum's area, there are some confusing ideas that they both are one and the same neurophysiologic process; however, this is not the case. Each is a separate process requiring different stimuli and evoking different responses. Fusion of only one object point in an otherwise formless visual field (Fig 5-8) can

occur, but this is inadequate as a stimulus for stereopsis. Fusion of a multitude of object points arranged on a horopter can occur, but stereopsis of these object points is impossible. For stereopsis to occur, the retina must be stimulated by at least two object points having a different proximal-distal relationship with each other in reference to the horopter (Fig 5-9). Furthermore, the retinal image disparity produced by these object points must be horizontal, since stereopsis does not occur in response to vertical or torsional retinal image disparity. But fusion of all disparate retinal images that result from object points within Panum's area occurs, no matter whether the image disparity is horizontal, vertical, or torsional. Thus, all disparate retinal images producing stereopsis are also fused, but not all disparate images that are fusible produce stereopsis; also, nondisparate retinal images are fusible, but never will such images produce stereopsis.

One additional vast difference between fusion and stereopsis is the motor component. Fusion has a motor component; stereopsis has none. Fusional vergence is the motor component of fusion, designed to reduce horizontal, vertical, and torsional disparity of the retinal image to the degree that fusion can be attained and/or maintained. By fusing, stereopsis also is gained if the horizontal retinal image disparity is present. Stereopsis, however, has no identifiable isolated motor component designed solely to achieve the proper retinal image disparity that produces stereopsis. For example, the ideal circumstance for fusion is total absence of image disparity, and the fusional vergence aligns the eyes toward this goal, even though Panum's area makes it unnecessary to absolutely achieve it. However, stereopsis requires horizontal image disparity, but no motor component serves this requirement in behalf of stereopsis. Stereopsis appreciation becomes more and more difficult as the quantity of fusible retinal image disparity is reduced, and minimal disparity evoking this perception is 10 to 14 seconds of arc. Although in many everyday seeing circumstances stereopsis would be enhanced by adjusting the eye alignment and increasing the horizontal image disparity, it cannot occur because no motor reflex exists to produce it.

Still another difference between fusion and stereopsis is their respective effectiveness for distal object points. The horizontal retinal image disparity required for stereopsis is produced by the horizontal separation of right and left retinas. A separation of only approximately 6 cm, this distance

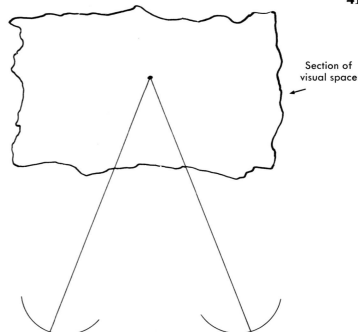

Fig 5-8. An isolated object point within a formless field projected onto corresponding retinal areas is fused, but there can be no appreciation of stereopsis.

Fig 5-9. Stereopsis requires at least two object points within Panum's area simultaneously stimulating the retina.

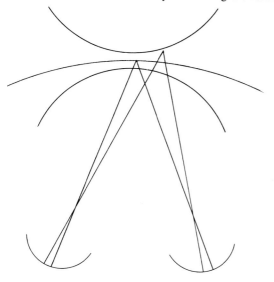

soon becomes inadequate to yield sufficient horizontal retinal image disparity to produce stereopsis as the viewing distance between object points and the eyes is increased. In 1838 Wheatstone wrote, "Although the accuracy of the stereoscopic sense is comparable with vernier acuity its range is comparatively limited. With the naked eye stereoscopic vision does not extend beyond 2000 feet. The radius of stereoscopic vision is about 7000 times the interpupillary baseline." With the teleostereoscope invented by Helmholtz in 1857, the effective baseline was extended by the use of right-angled prisms, with a proportionate increase in the stereoscopic vision. Prism binocular field glasses and stereoscopic range finders are constructed on this principle. In contrast to the limited range for stereopsis, fusion is equally effective for all ranges because the visual stimuli evoking it are not related to the interpupillary baseline.

Fusion and stereopsis serve different functions. Fusion localizes object points in a two-dimensional plane for the observer, while stereopsis localizes in the third dimension of depth. Hence, fusion and stereopsis differ not only in the visual stimuli required for their responses and the nature of their responses but also in their ultimate contribution to single binocular vision. They are quite different neurophysiologic entities, sharing only one component, ie, the visual stimuli that produce their responses arise from object points within Panum's area.

CENTRAL AND PERIPHERAL SINGLE BINOCULAR VISION

There are some peculiarities of the cortical function that, unrelated to the characteristic of the light stimulus, determine the nature of the single binocular vision.

Attention is a dominant factor in determining what is seen within the overall visual environment. During ordinary seeing one is conscious of visual material only within a relatively small area of the entire visual field: the area of conscious regard (Fig 5-10). There is no fixed measurement for this spatial area, but it is approximately 3° to 5° in diameter and usually projects onto the maximal resolving area of the retina. The object receiving maximal attention within this area of conscious attention usually is the object of regard as it is imaged on the fovea and its immediate surrounds. This means the cortex usually is attentive only to the image material projecting on the cones comprising the maculas.

Information supplied to the cortex from the visual field peripheral to the area of conscious regard (Fig 5-11) is usually processed at a subconscious level; this permits the subject to accurately maneuver about, maintaining attention to visual material within the area of conscious regard but oblivious to his general environment.

Central single binocular vision is cortical integration of the image projected onto each macula from the area of conscious regard (Fig 5-12). It receives high attention from the beholder and comprises the bulk of what one is visually aware of. Peripheral single binocular vision is an extramacular function that serves the visual space peripheral to the area of conscious regard. Although attention to this visual area is low, peripheral vision is of major importance for the subconscious orientation of the organism in his surroundings in space.

Single binocular vision may occur for all images on both the macular and extramacular regions of the two eyes, hence both central and peripheral single binocular vision may be present. But central single binocular vision is not invariably coexistent with peripheral single binocular vision. Peripheral single binocular vision frequently exists alone, without central single binocular vision, but the reverse is never true.

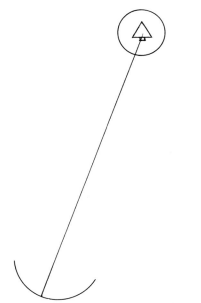

Fig 5-10. Area of conscious regard is limited to a few degrees.

Fig 5-11. Field of vision peripheral to area of conscious regard.

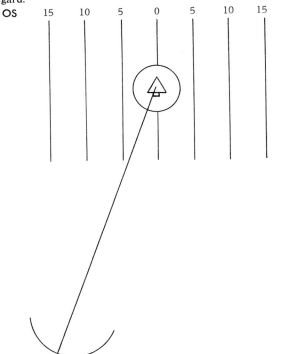

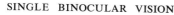

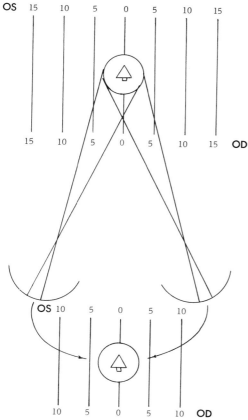

Fig 5-12. Central fusion is fusion of retinal sensations from visual stimuli within area of conscious regard.

TABLE 5-2. Components of Single Binocular Vision

	Central	Peripheral
Simultaneous perception	None	Excellent
Fusion	Limited*	Excellent
Stereopsis	Excellent	Limited†

* Sensory component of fusion is normal, but motor component is deficient.

† Stereoacuity is poor since the highly resolving maculas are not simultaneously functioning, a requisite for appreciating the minimal image disparity required for excellent stereoacuity.

Fig 5-13. Dissimilar targets viewed by each eye, either by allowing eyes to become exotropic or by inserting base-in prism before eyes so the intersection of lines of the X and the center of the horizontal line are superimposed. While fixating center of the X, the eyes no longer perceive the center of the horizontal line. Conversely, while seeing the center of the horizontal line, they lose the center of the X. The portions of both the X and the horizontal line that are projected onto rod-populated retina are simultaneously perceived. As the paper is tilted, the centers of the dissimilar targets move vertically apart. When both centers project onto rod-populated retina, both entire dissimilar targets are seen. (From Adler FH: Physiology of the Eye. St. Louis: Mosby, 1959.)

There are both anatomic and neurophysiologic differences between central and peripheral fusion. The central rod-free area of the retina identifies central fusion as one mediated entirely by cones. The cortical region receiving macular input is larger than the cortex representing all the extramacular retinal areas. The cones have a 1:1 cortical representation, compared to the pyramid arrangement of the neurons, starting with the rods, resulting in many rods being represented by one cortical cell. Possibly these anatomic differences create the conditions for different neurophysiology between central and peripheral fusion.

Dissimilarly contoured images, as alluded to previously in this chapter, are not simultaneously perceived by the central rod-free areas of the retinas, yet they are perceived by the extramacular portions of the retinas (Fig 5-13). Therefore, simultaneous perception is a function of single binocular vision confined to the extramacular retinal areas. It does not occur in central single binocular vision. Central single binocular vision has only two components, ie, fusion and stereopsis, whereas peripheral single binocular vision possesses all three, ie, simultaneous perception, fusion, and stereopsis (Table 5-2). This knowledge is essential in understanding the adaptations that occur in the single binocular vision of young people when they acquire strabismus.

The sensory aspect of fusion is equally good for both central and peripheral single binocular vision, but the motor aspect of fusion is very deficient in central and excellent in peripheral single binocular vision. Fusible, similarly contoured image material projected only onto the macular areas evokes very minimal fusional vergence amplitudes. These fusible targets must project onto the extramacular areas to produce a normal motor fusional response. The fusional vergence amplitudes of a person having only peripheral single binocular vision are just as good as those of his counterpart with central single binocular vision.

Stereopsis can be quantitated into the seconds of arc of retinal image disparity required to produce the perception, the minimal disparity that elicits the response. For very minimal quantities of retinal image disparity to be appreciated, the images must simultaneously project onto retinal areas having maximal resolving power. Since maximal resolving power occurs within the macular areas, the perception of stereopsis is obtainable for minimally disparate retinal images projecting on them that would not evoke stereopsis if they projected extramacularly. Peripheral single binocular vision provides gross stereopsis, but fine stereopsis is a product of central single binocular vision. Therefore, stereoacuity based on the least disparity in retinal images that produces stereopsis can be used for proving the presence of central single binocular vision. Figure 5-14 shows the Wirt Polaroid vectographic stereotest that presents varied quantities of horizontal retinal image disparity to the patient. Patients without central single binocular vision have an average stereoacuity of 200 seconds of arc but never better than 67 seconds of arc; the average person with central single binocular vision has an average stereoacuity of 24 seconds of arc and possibly as good as 14 seconds of arc (3).

ACQUISITION OF SINGLE BINOCULAR VISION

Single binocular vision apparently is a conditioned reflex. The requisites for its development are straight eyes (ideally from birth) and similar images presented to each retina. Congenitally strabismic patients do not have single binocular vision, but peripheral single binocular vision may develop after the strabismus is eliminated (4). There is

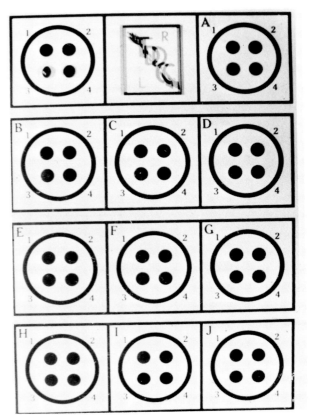

Fig 5-14. Wirt Polaroid vectograph test for stereoacuity, with test range between 14 and 1,000 seconds of arc.

some evidence that a higher percentage of those whose strabismus is eliminated at a very young age develop single binocular vision than those who are older when the strabismus is eliminated. It is impossible to declare the maximum age at which congenitally strabismic patients can develop single binocular vision after having their eyes straightened, but most clinicians believe that the maximum is 2 years of age (4–7). Grossly dissimilar images presented to each retina, such as occurs in high degrees of anisometropia or in disturbances of the clear media of one eye, preclude the development of single binocular vision, comparable to congenital strabismus.

The first clinical evidence of single binocular vision may be demonstrated at approximately 6 months of age by convergence of the eye in response to an 8△ base-out prism slipped in front of it. Once single binocular vision has developed, it will never be surrendered as long as both retinas are functioning and are able to be stimulated adequately with images. Children 10 years of age or less are able to make adaptations in the neurophysiology of single binocular vision so it may continue to function without symptoms despite acquired strabismus. Older children and adults are victims of annoying symptoms that never disappear if they acquire strabismus after the development of binocular vision.

REFERENCES

1. Worth C: Squint: Its Causes, Pathology, and Treatment. Philadelphia: Blakiston, 1908
2. Adler FH: Physiology of the Eye. St. Louis: Mosby, 1959
3. Parks MM: Stereoacuity as an indicator of bifixation. In Strabismus Symposium, Giessen. Basel Karger: August 1966, pp 258–260
4. Ing M, Costenbader FD, Parks MM, Albert DG: Early surgery for congenital esotropia. Am J Ophthalmol 61:1419, 1966
5. Parks MM: Early operations for strabismus. Transactions of the First Congress of the International Strabismological Association. London, 1971, pp 29–36
6. von Noorden GK, Isaza A, Parks ME: Surgical treatment of congenital esotropia. Trans Am Acad Ophthalmol Otolaryngol 76:1465, 1972
7. Taylor DM: Is congenital esotropia functionally curable? Trans Am Ophthalmol Soc 70:529, 1972

6

Alignment

the ability of the curved corneal surface to reflect an examining light, the dissimilar image tests which are based on the patient's response to diplopia produced by converting an isolated object of regard into different images on each retina, and the dissimilar target tests which are based on the patient's response to the dissimilar images created by each eye viewing a different target.

COVER TESTS. Since the cover tests are based on the fixation ability of the eye, that must first be assessed. Patients without fixation ability in each eye (eccentric fixation) are unable to have eye alignment checked by cover tests. Also, the patient's accommodation must be controlled by using an appropriate target. An accommodative target is a small target designed to control the patient's accommodation if his response supplies clear vision; this target is required during the cover test.

Cover-Uncover. The patient's right eye is covered while he fixates a series of distant accommodative targets. After two to three seconds, the right eye is uncovered and the left eye covered. When covering one eye, the examiner's attention is directed to the opposite, uncovered eye, looking for movement of this eye. An absence of movement of an eye when the other eye is covered (Fig 6-1), occurring in both eyes, means that the patient does not have a heterotropia, but it does not differentiate between orthophoria and heterophoria. The alternate cover test is required to make this differentiation.

Alternate Cover. The basic principle of this test is to prevent fusion for the duration of the test. This is accomplished by constantly maintaining a cover over one or the other eye, shifting it swiftly from eye to eye while the examiner looks for movement of the uncovered eye as it assumes fixation (Fig 6-2). The rapid shift applies only to the speed of movement of the cover and not to the duration it is held before the eye; in fact, the examiner should maintain the cover over each eye for two or three seconds before rapidly shifting it. No movement of either eye indicates orthophoria. The patient whose eye moves on alternate cover has either a heterophoria or heterotropia. Differentiation between the two requires the cover-uncover test, since there is movement to neither cover-uncover nor alternate cover testing in orthophoria. The direction of the shift identifies the type of heterophoria or heterotropia. A temporal horizontal shift is esophoria or esotropia, a nasal shift is exophoria or exotropia, and right or left hyperphoria or hypertropia is the movement of the right or the left eye downward. If both eyes make movements downward it is called

PRIMARY POSITION

Classification

I. Orthophoria. The eyes are perfectly aligned, and no deviation occurs even when the fusion reflex is disrupted.

II. Heterophoria and Heterotropia. Misalignment compensated for by the fusion reflex keeps the deviation in heterophoria latent. Manifest misalignment is heterotropia.

    A. Horizontal

        1. Esophoria or esotropia: convergent deviation of the visual axes

        2. Exophoria or exotropia: divergent deviation of the visual axes

    B. Vertical

        1. Right hyperphoria or hypertropia: right visual axis is deviated upward compared to the left

        2. Left hyperphoria or hypertropia: left visual axis is deviated upward compared to the right

    C. Torsional

        1. Incyclophoria or incyclotropia: superior poles of the corneas are tipped medially

        2. Excyclophoria or excyclotropia: superior poles of the corneas are tipped temporally

Determination

The methods used to determine the eye alignment in the primary position are varied and multiple. No single test invariably assesses the alignment accurately in all patients.

There are four basic types of alignment tests: the various cover tests which depend on the fixation reflex, the corneal reflex tests which are based on

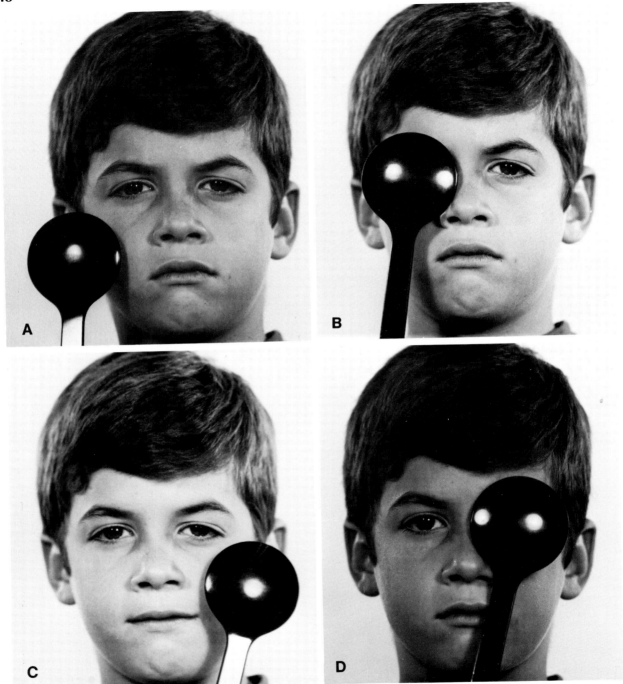

Fig 6-1. Cover-uncover test. **A.** Examiner observes left eye as he prepares to cover right eye. **B.** Right eye is covered. **C.** Right eye is uncovered. Right eye is observed as preparation is made to cover left eye. **D.** Left eye is covered.

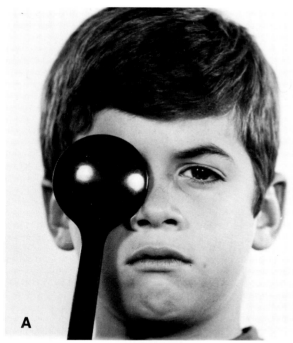

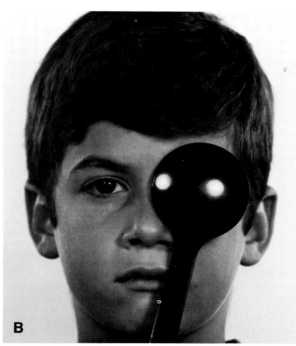

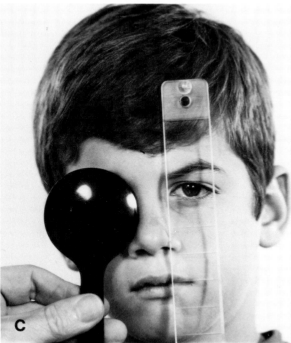

Fig 6-2. Alternate cover test. Cover before right eye (**A**) is rapidly transferred to left eye (**B**) as examiner observes right eye for any shift it may make to establish fixation. Alternately transferring the cover from eye to eye while observing the uncovered eye discloses any heterodeviation that may be present, provided each eye can centrally fixate. **C.** Introducing a prism before one eye allows measurement of the heterodeviation (prism and alternate cover test).

dissociated double hyperphoria or hypertropia (alternating sursumduction). This type of deviation not compensated for by the fusion reflex is referred to as dissociated double hypertropia (see chapter titled Dissociated Hyperdeviations).

Having identified a heterodeviation, the next step is to measure the quantity of misalignment by neutralizing the shift with prism power. The prism is held in the examiner's left hand in front of the patient's right eye. The examiner's right hand handles the alternate cover. The prism or prism powers are adjusted until the motion of the eyes on alternate cover is eliminated (Fig 6-2, *C*). Base-out prisms are used to compensate for an eso-deviation, base-in for an exodeviation, base-down before the right eye for a right hyperdeviation, and base-up for a left hyperdeviation. Horizontal and vertical prism powers can be combined if loose prisms are used. A prism bar is handy, but it does not lend itself to neutralizing combined horizontal and vertical deviations nor is it sufficient to compensate for horizontal deviations greater than 40Δ or vertical deviations greater than 25△. The loose prisms must be combined for larger deviations. Vertical deviations seldom exceed 25△, but horizontal tropias greater than 40△ are very common. The most convenient way for the examiner to hold combined horizontal prisms is not to superimpose them before one eye but instead to grasp the horizontal prisms either apex-to-apex (esotropia) or base-to-base (exotropia) between the thumb and index finger of his left hand, allowing his finger and thumb to cup around the patient's right eye, with one prism being positioned before each eye. The area of contact between the apexes or bases then is in the midline in front of the patient's nose. Prisms cannot neutralize cyclodeviations.

Simultaneous Prism and Cover. This test is useful in a patient having a small-angle heterotropia, commonly encountered in esotropes. The simultaneous prism and cover test is an attempt to measure the actual heterotropia angle present under normal seeing conditions while both eyes are uncovered. As the fixating eye is covered, a prism of known power is slipped simultaneously before the opposite eye with its base in the appropriate direction to compensate for the heterotropia. No movement occurs as the eye behind the prism takes up fixation when the prism power selected equals the heterotropia angle. This measurement is important because of a prevalent condition known as the monofixation syndrome. Some patients having this syndrome are small-angle heterotropes; among these there are some who reduce their larger fusion-free angle (as determined by alternate cover) to a smaller angle during normal seeing conditions. For example, the esotropia may measure 14△ by alternate cover, but the simultaneous prism and cover may reveal 4△ esotropia that the patient maintains with both eyes open.

CORNEAL REFLEX TESTS. Studying the reflection of an examining light provides information regarding the alignment of the eyes in patients who cannot cooperate sufficiently to perform the alternate cover test or who lack fixation ability due to amblyopia. Four techniques may be employed using this principle. The Hirschberg test grossly estimates the angle of strabismus according to the degree of displacement away from the pupillary center at which the examiner views the corneal reflection in the deviated eye. A second method is the Krimsky test, which entails introducing prisms before either one or both eyes in order to center the corneal reflections in the pupil of each. The third is a perimeter method, and the fourth is a major amblyoscope method. In the latter two methods, the alignment is read on the machine at the point the corneal reflections are centered in the pupils. The unit of strabismic deviation according to the Hirschberg and perimeter tests is degrees; for the Krimsky and major amblyoscope tests it is prism diopters.

Hirschberg Method. A light reflected in the deviated eye nearer the pupillary center than the margin is estimated to be a 5° to 6° squint, at the pupillary margin is 12° to 15°, midway between pupillary margin and limbus is 25°, at the limbus is 45° to 60°, and beyond the limbus is 60° to 80° (Fig 6-3). Roughly, each 1-mm deviation of light reflex away from the proper position indicates 7° of squint.

Krimsky Method. The corneal reflections of the examining light are compared in regard to the location of the pupil in each eye. Dissimilar positions are indicative of strabismus. By placing proper prism power before either one or both eyes simultaneously, the reflection can be similarly positioned (Fig 6-4); this is a direct reading of the estimated squint angle.

Perimeter Method. The perimeter method requires the patient to steadily fixate the zero mark on the perimeter with the preferred eye while the examiner moves an examining light and his aligning eye together along the back side of the perimeter arc. At the point on the arc that the corneal reflection of the light appears located in the pupillary center of the deviated eye, the perimeter arc marking measures the squint angle in degrees (Fig 6-5).

Major Amblyoscope Method. The amblyoscope is basically a refined haploscopic device which originally consisted of a median septum between the two eyes plus angled mirrors that reflected separate targets into each eye. The present-day

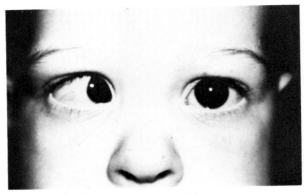

Fig 6-3. Hirschberg corneal reflex test.

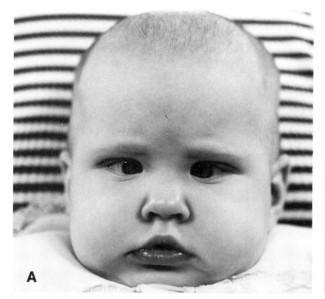
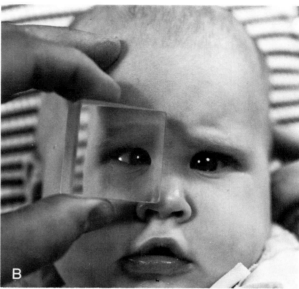

Fig 6-4. Krimsky corneal reflex test. **A.** Congenital esotropic infant. **B.** Measuring esotropic angle.

Fig 6-5. Perimeter corneal reflex test.

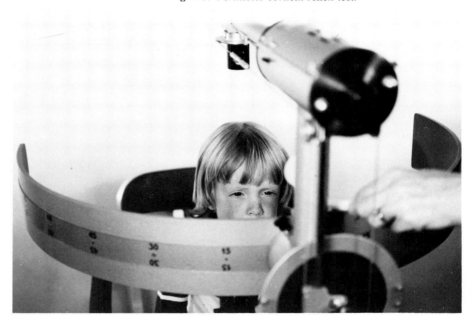

amblyoscope, instead of using a septum and mirrors, has a separate tube for each eye with a housing at the distal end of each tube in which it is possible to insert an assortment of targets to be visualized individually by each eye. Further refinements, such as separate illumination of each target that is capable of being varied by rheostats and

tubes that are mounted so they can be deflected in any plane and the quantity of deflection read directly from calibrated scales, make this instrument a major amblyoscope. Adjusting the tubes so that the corneal reflections of the illumination within the target housing is centered in each pupil (Fig 6-6) gives the examiner a direct reading of the patient's

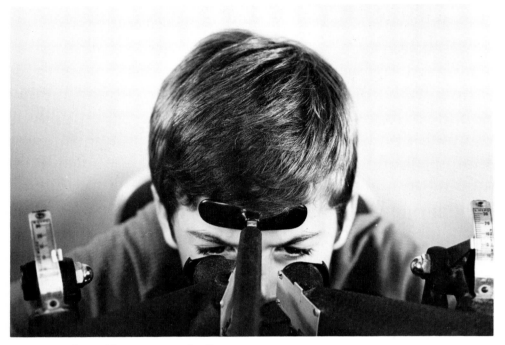

Fig 6-6. Major amblyoscope corneal reflex test.

Fig 6-7. Angle kappa.

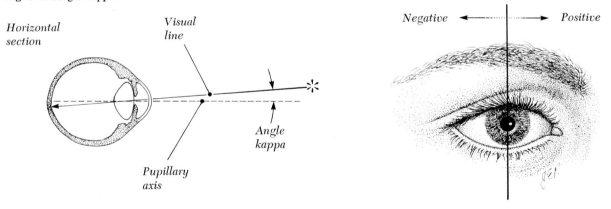

misalignment from the instrument's scales. Regardless of which corneal reflex technique is used, consideration must be given to the angle kappa. Since the fixation axis does not usually accurately penetrate the center of the pupil, the corneal reflex of the light being fixated is off-center. The angle formed by an imaginary perpendicular line through the true pupillary center and the fixation axis is the angle kappa (Fig 6-7). A nasal angle kappa is designated as positive and a temporal angle as negative. It can be measured by any one of the above methods.

Both horizontal and vertical misalignments can be studied by the corneal reflex methods, but the examiner is unable to use these methods in the study of the cyclodeviations.

DISSIMILAR IMAGES TESTS. The same fixation target which is simultaneously presented to each eye is converted into dissimilar images on the right and the left retina for the purpose of making fusion difficult or impossible. The Maddox rod test and the red glass test are two commonly used testing methods based on making the one object of regard

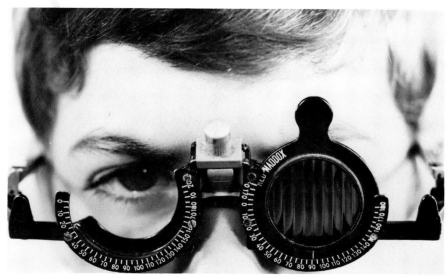

Fig 6-8. Maddox rod positioned in trial frame for investigation of vertical deviation.

project as dissimilar retinal images. Both tests are of value in assessing alignment only if the status of the retinal correspondence is known.

Maddox rod. The Maddox rod is a ribbed lens, the "washboard" appearance of which converts a spot of light into a streak. The streak is seen by the patient 90° away from the axes of the multiple cylinders. The rod is placed before one eye as the other eye continues to fixate the small spot source of light; a streak is seen to pass through the light if there is no deviation in the plane being tested. A horizontal streak (ribbing of the Maddox rod is vertical) checks vertical plane alignment (Fig 6-8) and a vertical streak (ribbing of the Maddox rod is horizontal) checks the horizontal plane alignment. If the streak appears displaced away from the light, a misalignment exists. Whether the misalignment is a phoria or a tropia cannot be determined, since fusion is precluded in this test. In the horizontal plane testing, a homonymous diplopia indicates esodeviation and heteronymous diplopia indicates exodeviation. In the vertical plane testing, the streak seen by the hyperdeviated eye appears lower than the light and vice versa for the hypodeviated eye. Prisms are used to eliminate the horizontal or vertical diplopia, yielding a direct measure of the deviation if the retinal correspondence is normal. Cyclodeviations can be checked by placing a Maddox rod, preferably one red and the other white, before each eye at the same axis setting for each eye. If the axes of the two Maddox rods are set at 90 (Fig 6-9), the red and white streaks appear on different axes in cyclodeviation. By adjustment

in the axis settings of the two Maddox rods they are made to appear parallel; thus the degree of cyclodeviation can be determined.

Red Filter. While the patient fixates a small spot source of light, a red lens is placed before one of his eyes (Fig 6-10). This test accomplishes the same thing as the Maddox rod in the horizontal and vertical deviations, but it is of no value in investigating cyclodeviations. It is less likely to disrupt fusion than the Maddox rod since only the color and the intensity of the images are made dissimilar while the contour of the images in the right and the left eye remains the same. The patient can fuse the white and the red light into a "pink" light. Prisms are used to eliminate the horizontal or vertical diplopia, yielding a direct measure of the deviation if the retinal correspondence is normal.

DISSIMILAR TARGET TESTS. A number of different techniques for evaluating alignment are based on the presentation of different targets to the right and the left eye while the patient adjusts the projection device to superimpose the dissimilar images. If the retinal correspondence is normal, the point at which the images appear superimposed provides a direct reading of the patient's alignment. The two most widely used methods employing this principle are the Lancaster red-green projectors and the major amblyoscope.

Lancaster Red-Green Projectors. One projector shines a red target and the other a green target on

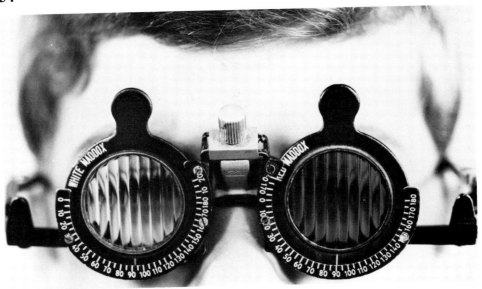

Fig 6-9. Double maddox rod.

Fig 6-10. Red filter in trial frame.

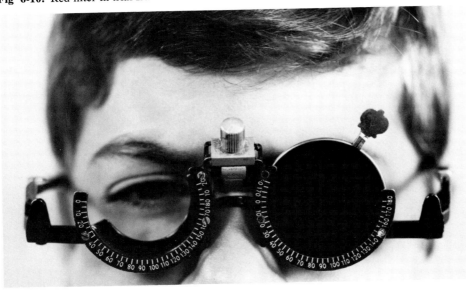

a white screen marked with a grid calibrated in prism diopters; the screen is 1 meter from the patient. The targets, of similar contour and intensity, are viewed by the patient with red-green spectacles (red filter before one eye and green before the other). The patient adjusts the targets so they appear superimposed (Fig 6-11), thus affording a direct reading of any deviation. Horizontal, vertical, and torsional deviations are well revealed since the targets are linear, 2 to 3 cm in length.

Major Amblyoscope. The patient views the dissimilar targets which are simultaneously deposited in the housing of each tube and adjusts them so that the images, eg, bird and cage, car and garage, fish and bowl, are superimposed (Fig 5-7, *A*). If the retinal correspondence is normal, the horizontal, vertical, and torsional deviations are read directly from the scales on the instrument that record the deflections of the tubes away from zero in these three planes. Furthermore, the illumination of the tubes can be alternately flashed on and off,

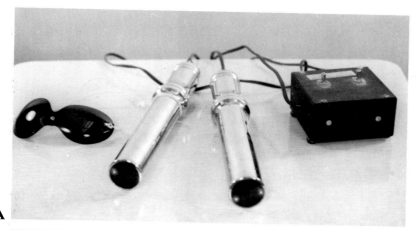

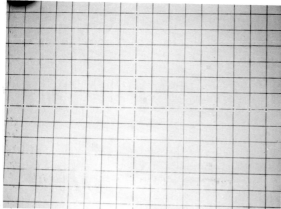

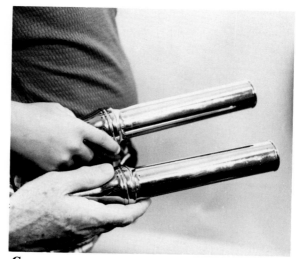

Fig 6-11. Lancaster red-green projectors. **A.** Projectors with red-green spectacles. **B.** Grid screen. **C.** While looking through a red filter before one eye and a green filter before the other the patient attempts to project his green target so that it appears superimposed upon the red target projected by the examiner. A direct reading of the heterodeviation is made from the separation of the targets as they project upon the screen.

allowing only one eye to view the target at a time. By observing the movement of the eyes as they fixate first one and then the other target, the examiner can adjust the tubes so as to eliminate all movement (Fig 6-12). This, in effect, is an alternate cover test; however, instead of using prisms to measure the quantity of deviation, it is recorded by the scales on the instrument.

With the exception of testing methods using the major amblyoscope, primary position alignment may be investigated both while the head is erect or when it is tilted to either shoulder. The purpose of testing the alignment in the primary position with the head tilted is to study the effect of the utricular reflex in cyclovertical muscle deviations. The head is rotated about the coronal axis for 60°

toward either shoulder, and the alignment is checked by cover tests, corneal reflex tests, dissimilar image tests, or the Lancaster red-green projectors.

SECONDARY POSITIONS

The three secondary positions are near fixation, cardinal positions, and midline position.

NEAR FIXATION

The purpose of investigating near fixation is to study the effect that the convergence associated with accommodation (synkinetic near reflex) has on the alignment of the eyes. Therefore, only the horizontal plane (esodeviations and exodeviations) is of significance; the vertical plane (hyperdeviations) and torsional plane (cyclodeviations) are irrelevant.

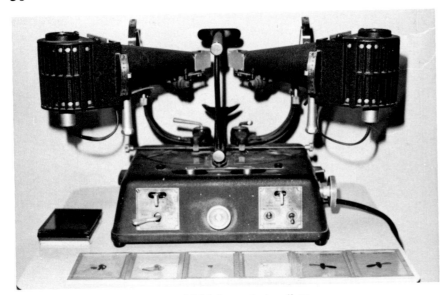

Fig 6-12. Major amblyoscope. Multiple controls allow variable illumination to each target housing, illumination of the tube to be alternately flashed on and off, and adjustments to be made for the patient's interpupillary distance and horizontal, vertical, and torsional plane deviation that is read directly from scales.

Classification

The classifications of near fixation are as follows:

1. Normal. The distant (primary position) and near position alignment are comparable.
2. Abnormal. The distant and near position alignment are incomparable.
   a. Convergence excess: greater esodeviation at near than at distance
   b. Convergence insufficiency: greater exodeviation at near than at distance
   c. Divergence excess: greater exodeviation at distance than at near
   d. Divergence insufficiency: greater esodeviation at distance than at near

Determination

The near point usually chosen to study the near alignment is 0.33 meter from the eyes. The test must be conducted in such a manner that the accommodation is stimulated. This requires that the target have fine pattern detail such as is found in small pictures, Snellen letters, numbers, and print. A small muscle light does not satisfy this requirement; therefore, for this measurement it is not used.

Since a light source is an unsatisfactory target for testing the near position, then the corneal reflex tests, dissimilar image tests, and the Lancaster projector tests are excluded for near testing. The only satisfactory tests for the near position are the cover test (cover-uncover, alternate cover, and simultaneous prism and cover) and the major amblyoscope if targets demanding foveal vision are used. To stimulate accommodation, −3.00 lenses are inserted before each eye, simulating a test performed at 0.33 meter.

CARDINAL POSITIONS

The purpose of studying these six positions is to compare the prime mover of the one eye for each of these positions with the comparable prime mover of the other eye (Fig 2-4). Only the horizontal and vertical planes are tested; the torsional plane is disregarded.

Classification

The classifications of the cardinal positions are as follows:

1. Normal. The horizontal and the vertical plane alignment are orthophoric in all six cardinal positions.
2. Abnormal. There is a horizontal and/or a vertical plane misalignment in one or all of the six cardinal positions.
   a. Concomitant. The deviation is identical in all positions.
      (1) Horizontal
         (a) Esodeviation
         (b) Exodeviation
      (2) Vertical
         (a) Right hyperdeviation
         (b) Left hyperdeviation

b. Nonconcomitant. The deviation varies in different gaze positions.
    (1) Horizontal
        (a) Esodeviation
        (b) Exodeviation
    (2) Vertical
        (a) Right hyperdeviation
        (b) Left hyperdeviation

Determination

Horizontal deviations are studied by comparing the alignment in approximately 30° right gaze and 30° left gaze. Vertical deviations are examined by measuring the alignment in not only 30° right and left gaze, but also in 30° up and right, down and right, up and left, and down and left. All measurements can be done at either distant fixation (6 meters) or near fixation (0.33 meter), it being unnecessary to do both. The particular tests may be cover tests (cover-uncover, alternate cover), corneal reflex tests (Hirschberg method, Krimsky method, perimeter method), dissimilar image tests (Maddox rod, red filter), or dissimilar target tests (Lancaster red-green projectors). The major amblyoscope study is performed with the eyes in the straight-ahead position; therefore, this technique cannot be used for investigating alignment in the cardinal positions.

The cover tests, dissimilar image tests, and Lancaster red-green projector tests may be performed either by maintaining the patient's head in the same position while the targets are moved or by maintaining the targets in the same position while the patient's head is turned and tipped in various directions with the eyes continuing to fixate the target.

Some nonconcomitant deviations measure differently in the primary position, depending on whether the right or the left eye is fixating. When fixating with the eye that has normal muscles (primary deviation) the deviation is less than when fixating with the eye having the paretic muscle (secondary deviation); therefore, the secondary deviation exceeds the primary deviation. Apparently more innervation is required to drive the involved eye into the fixating primary position than to drive the uninvolved. Since the paretic muscle and its yoke receive equal innervational input and the normal muscle can move its eye much further than can the paretic muscle, the increased innervation fed into the paretic muscle to align the eye for primary position fixation results in the normal yoke muscle overdeviating the uninvolved eye.

The best way to mask the nonconcomitant deviation is to maintain the eyes in the gaze position which has the least deviation. This results in compensatory head posture. For example, a patient having a palsied right lateral rectus masks the abduction deficiency by maintaining his right eye in adduction; in order to see straight ahead while his eyes are in left gaze, his face is turned right. Compensatory postures of the eyes and head are simple in the case of an isolated palsy of a horizontal rectus, but this is not so for the other muscles. A simple compensatory elevation or depression of the eyes solves only part of the diplopia problem caused by an isolated, underacting vertical rectus or oblique. One must remember that the vertical action of these muscles is in either adduction or abduction, and in the direction of gaze opposite to the field of vertical action there is torsional action. In the primary position there is a combined cyclovertical action. There is a combined torsional and vertical diplopia in the primary position, becoming more torsional and less vertical in one direction of gaze and the reverse in the opposite direction of gaze. For example, the vertical diplopia caused by a paretic right superior oblique is alleviated by abducting the right eye. Although abduction is out of the depressor field of action of the superior oblique, it is in the position for maximal intorsion. Consequently, solving the vertical diplopia by assuming a horizontal gaze and compensatory turning of the face worsens the torsional diplopia. The reverse horizontal gaze and face turn diminishes the torsional diplopia but increases the vertical diplopia. This patient does two things to rid himself of the cyclovertical diplopia. The head is tilted to the left and the eyes are elevated. The latter causes chin depression (Fig 19-6). The left head tilt, by way of the utricular reflex, and the elevation of the eyes combine to mask the weak right eye intortor and depressor, since each results in inhibitory innervation to the right superior oblique. Isolated cylovertical muscle palsies, then, are associated with the combined compensatory head postures: chin elevation or depression and head tilt. The compensatory head posture caused by an ocular motility defect is responsible for the descriptive term "ocular torticollis." However, palsy of an extraocular muscle is not the only ocular motility defect that causes ocular torticollis. Patients with congenital nystagmus frequently have ocular torticollis, carrying their head in a horizontal, a vertical, or a torsional plane to improve their vision by reducing the excursion of their uncontrollable oscillatory eye movements. A number of ocular motility defects other than palsy of an extraocular muscle that frequently are associated with ocular torticollis are included in the next section of the chapter.

MIDLINE POSITIONS

Both horizontal and vertical plane deviations are studied in the up and down midline positions.

Classification

The classifications of midline positions are as follows:

1. Normal. The horizontal and the vertical plane alignment are orthophoric in both straight upgaze and downgaze.
2. Abnormal. A horizontal and/or a vertical plane misalignment is present in the upgaze position and/or the downgaze position.
   a. Horizontal
      (1) A pattern
      (2) V pattern
   b. Vertical
      (1) Double elevator palsy
      (2) Fibrosis of a vertical rectus muscle
      (3) Myopathy due to thyroid disease
      (4) Adherence syndrome

   (a) Following fracture of orbital floor
   (b) Following surgery of extraocular muscles
   (c) Brown's syndrome

Determination

The cover tests, the corneal reflex tests, the dissimilar image tests, and the dissimilar target tests are used to study the midline positions of 30° straight above the primary position and 30° below it. It is possible to use the major amblyoscope in performing the midline position analysis.

Both A or V horizontal deviations and vertical deviations may be minimized by positioning the eyes a certain number of degrees above or below the primary position, thus allowing the patient to obtain binocular vision. The chin is then raised or lowered to offset this compensatory eye position, resulting in a compensatory head posture. Therefore, ocular deviations that are influenced by upgaze or downgaze may cause an ocular torticollis characterized by either chin elevation or depression.

7

Vergences

The vergences are reflexes, an integral factor in strabismus. They are the principal cause of concomitant deviations as well as the principal compensator, masking the deviation contained in a phoria rather than allowing it to become an overt tropia.

The vergence eye movements are produced by a group of compound reflexes, only two of which are identifiable because they are measurable; these are fusional vergence and accommodative convergence. The fusional vergences are optomotor reflexes designed to improve and maintain the alignment of the eyes so that similar retinal images project on corresponding retinal areas, a requirement for single binocular vision that utilizes normal retinal correspondence. The accommodative convergence is a reflex linking convergence automatically to accommodation and supplying the most economical innervating method for achieving proper alignment simultaneously with a change in the dioptric power of the lens as attention shifts rapidly between a remote point and a proximal point. Another vergence reflex, or perhaps other vergence reflexes, influences the alignment but remains ill-defined and not measurable; this unidentifiable entity which exerts vergence influence on the alignment makes up the tonic vergence.

ACCOMMODATIVE CONVERGENCE

The ciliary musculature contracts on the arrival of impulses at its myoneural junctions. The accommodative response is graded according to the quantity of impulses arriving. The degree of innervation dispatched to the ciliary muscles is associated with comparable gradations of innervation to the medial rectus and the sphincter pupillae. The combination of these three separate motor innervations producing the response of accommodation, convergence, and miosis is called the synkinetic near response. Normally the innervation proceeds to the respective muscles supplying these functions according to a ratio that permits relatively clear vision and approximate bifixation. Since convergence and miosis are also responses within other reflex systems, their particular responses to a near stimulus are designated as accommodative convergence and pupillary constriction to near stimulus. Accommodation differs from convergence and miosis in that it occurs only within the framework of the synkinetic near reaction.

The following four stimuli produce the synkinetic near response:

1. A blurred retinal image focused posterior to the plane of the retina. Regardless of whether the object projecting as a blurred image is far away or near, accommodation is applied. Accompanying the accommodation are the other two components of the synkinetic near response.
2. Bitemporal disparate retinal images. Accommodative convergence is used to reduce the bitemporal disparity in some patients similar to the way fusional convergence is used. Bitemporal retinal image disparity alone is enough to initiate the near response in some patients with exodeviations. Often a synkinetic near response to the bitemporal sharply focused retinal images occurs in the young exodeviating emmetrope even while fixating at a distance.
3. Awareness of near. A psycho-optic influence reflexly causes the subject to put forth the synkinetic response while attentive to proximal points in space. The opposite, awareness of far, causes relaxation of the synkinetic near response while the patient is attentive to remote points in space. The subject induced to respond counter to these psycho-optic drives, ie, to relax the synkinetic near activity while looking at a near point through plus lenses or to stimulate this activity while looking at a far point through minus lenses, gives only a fraction of what the total response would be were he allowed to respond naturally in conformity with the awareness of near and far influences. Recognizing their inability to prevent all convergence during measurement of alignment at near positions while the subject looks through plus lenses, many investigators have labeled this inevitable convergence response "proximal convergence." Clinically, a similar situation has been recognized while doing simulated distant alignment

measurements on instruments requiring near fixation through plus lenses. Invariably, such simulated distant measurements are more convergent than true distant measurements. However, such terms as "proximal convergence" and "instrument convergence" create a concept that these are separate entities within the spectrum of vergences rather than mere findings produced by the unnatural stimulation of the synkinetic near response.

4. Voluntary convergence. The synkinetic near activities usually occur at a subconscious level, as do reflexes. However, there is one outstanding exception. The synkinetic near activities that occur in response to a conscious desire to maximally converge the eyes are not reflex; this is voluntary convergence and is produced by fixating an imaginary near point. Associated with the convergence response are accommodation and miosis. Thus, voluntary convergence is a willed, forceful thrust of the entire spectrum of synkinetic near activities.

The accommodation and accommodative convergence components of the synkinetic near response are in perfect balance when each produces the satisfactory adjustments needed for clear vision and fusion over a wide range of fixation distances. If these activities are in proper relation, then the ratio of accommodative convergence to accommodation (AC/A) is normal. An abnormal AC/A is characterized by either a deficiency or an excess of accommodative convergence associated with each unit of accommodation; thus, the resulting abnormal ratio is either a low AC/A or a high AC/A.

NORMAL AC/A

The normal AC/A in children is pliable, an attribute that allows adjustments in uncorrected myopia and exodeviation.

The uncorrected myope tends to adjust the AC/A to a high ratio in order to obtain the maximal accommodative convergence and the deficient accommodation required for near vision. This compensation assists the myope to enjoy near binocularity. After the patient wears glasses for near vision for a few weeks, the high AC/A reverts to normal since it is no longer needed.

The young child with exodeviation tends to have a high AC/A which permits him to compensate maximally for the deviation and the bitemporal retinal image disparity it causes. After the exodeviation is corrected with surgery the ratio reverts toward normal since the high AC/A is no longer needed.

The normal ratio is influenced by certain drugs that alter the AC/A as long as they are present; however, when the drugs are withdrawn the AC/A reverts to the premedication level. The normal ratio is altered by parasympathomimetic and parasympatholytic drugs instilled into the eyes. Miotics potentiate the transmission of acetylcholine across the myoneural junction, allowing innervation to the ciliary muscle to produce a contraction greater than normal. This in turn results in a greater dioptric power change in the molding of the lens. However, associated with the innervation to the ciliary muscles is the same amount of innervation to the medial recti. Since the miotic has no effect on these muscles, there is no change in the quantity of convergence this amount of innervation produces. Consequently, the miotic alters the AC/A so that the response is more accommodation associated with an unchanged amount of accommodative convergence, ie, the miotic lowers the AC/A.

Weak cycloplegics partially prevent innervation arriving at the myoneural junction of the ciliary musculature from producing the expected dioptric increase in the refractive power of the lens. This is due to the reduction in the motor units firing in the ciliary musculature since the cycloplegia competes with the motor end-plates for the acetylcholine. Yet, the innervation simultaneously dispatched to the medial recti produces the normal convergence. The result is that the cycloplegic diminishes the accommodation response without changing the accommodative convergence, ie, the cycloplegic raises the AC/A.

ABNORMAL AC/A

An abnormal AC/A may be either a high or a low ratio. A high AC/A causes more convergence for near fixation than for distance fixation, with the actual difference between them being determined by the severity of the AC/A abnormality, which may vary from slight to marked. A high AC/A may occur in a patient with orthophoric eyes for distance fixation as well as in the patient with an esodeviation or an exodeviation. The patient with a high AC/A who is either orthophoric or esodeviated for distance was described by Duane (1) as having a convergence excess. The patient with a high AC/A with exodeviation at distance has a divergence excess (1).

The high AC/A is invariably the etiologic factor causing the convergence excess, and in this setting the high AC/A is primary, ie, it is primarily defective and not a secondary change in a normal AC/A. Depending on the refraction of the patient and the severity of this primarily abnormal AC/A, the eyes are straight, esophoric, or esotropic at distance, but regardless of the distant alignment, the esodeviation is invariably greater at near fixation. However, the high AC/A in the exotrope with divergence excess usually is an altered normal ratio that exercised its attribute of pliability, becoming a high ratio to help offset the exodeviation. Yet, the primarily defective high AC/A can occur in any type of patient, even an exotrope. It is possible that the patient with divergence excess may have either a high ratio that evolved from a normal one or a primarily abnormal high ratio, although the latter occurs infrequently. Most importantly, the primarily abnormal high AC/A is unpliable, unlike the normal AC/A. Surgically aligning the exodeviated eyes in a patient with divergence excess whose high AC/A is primarily defective results in a persistent esodeviation at near fixation, whereas the preoperative high AC/A adapted from a normal one promptly returns to normal postoperatively, nullifying any trend to near esotropia.

The primarily defective high AC/A that causes convergence excess tends to improve after the patient reaches 7 years of age. Miotics normalize the high AC/A but only while the drug is used; the miotic produces no permanent change in the AC/A. Surgery on the horizontal recti may improve the high AC/A somewhat; the greater the severity of the high AC/A, the greater is the effect of surgery on the ratio. There is no orthoptic technique that can improve the high AC/A.

A low AC/A causes less convergence for near fixation than for distance fixation, with the actual difference between them being determined by the severity of the AC/A abnormality, which may vary from slight to marked. A low AC/A may occur in a patient with orthophoric eyes for distance fixation as well as in a patient with esodeviation or exodeviation. The patient with a low AC/A who is either orthophoric or exodeviated for distance was described by Duane as having convergence insufficiency (1). The patient with a low AC/A and esodeviation at distance has a divergence insufficiency.

The low AC/A in convergence insufficiency is a primarily defective ratio that never improves with age. Although weak cycloplegics temporarily improve the low AC/A, this is of no practical value since the blurred vision and asthenopia produce symptoms more disturbing than those caused by the low AC/A. Neither surgery of the horizontal recti nor orthoptics improve the low AC/A in convergence insufficiency.

The low AC/A in divergence insufficiency is a relatively rare clinical entity. A very few esodeviated patients who fuse at near fixation but who are either esotropic or have a larger esophoria at distance have been studied; however, surgery has not been performed in a sufficient number to determine if there is a trend for the low AC/A to improve after the distance esodeviation is eliminated. Consequently, it is not known whether a low AC/A is the adjusted normal pliable AC/A that evolved to help offset the esotropia or whether it is a primarily defective unpliable ratio that just happens to occur in a small-angle esodeviation.

CLINICAL INVESTIGATION OF AC/A

Two simple methods of clinically investigating the AC/A are used extensively; however, regardless of which is used, the accommodation must be controlled while the study is conducted. Corrective lenses control the accommodation if the patient is other than emmetropic. Also, small-detailed fixating targets should be used rather than muscle lights. Prism and alternate cover measurements are made while the patient accommodates two different amounts. This enables the amount of convergence associated with accommodation to be evaluated.

One method of selecting the two separate quantities of accommodation for the patient is the distance-near measurements method, which alters the fixation distance. The most practical fixation distances are 6 meters and 0.33 meter. A normal AC/A is indicated by similar prism and alternate cover measurements at these two fixation points; dissimilar measurements indicate an abnormal ratio (Table 7-1).

The other method of selecting the two separate quantities of accommodation for the patient is the lens gradient method, which maintains the same fix-

TABLE 7-1. AC/A as Determined by Prism and Alternate Cover Measurements

	At 6 Meters	At 0.33 Meter
Normal ratio		
	Orthophoria	Orthophoria
	ET* = 30	ET = 30
	XT* = 30	XT = 30
Abnormal ratio		
High AC/A		
	Orthophoria	ET = 30
	ET = 30	ET = 60
	XT = 30	Orthophoria
Low AC/A		
	Orthophoria	XT = 15
	ET = 30	ET = 15
	XT = 30	XT = 45

* ET, esotropia; XT = exotropia.

ation distance while altering the accommodation with lenses. For example, 0.33 meter is used as the fixation distance, and prism and alternate cover measurements are performed first while the patient looks through +3.00 spheres and then without the lenses. Although the +3.00 spheres are a stimulus to relax the accommodation, the response is less than the stimulus because of awareness of near. Consequently, the values obtained by the lens gradient method in a patient with a normal AC/A are less than those obtained by the distance-near measurement method. Abnormal AC/A, whether high or low, is detected by either method, but the absolute values do not correspond. The lens gradient method is the preference of the researcher in this field, and the distance-near measurement method is the choice of the clinician. Usually, as the student first encounters the AC/A, he wants absolute figures delineating the range of normal. Accommodative convergence in prism diopters related to A in diopters by the lens gradient method is usually in the range of 3.7 to 4.2 in the normal person. However, this absolute figure for the lens gradient method is not particularly meaningful when the student evaluates patients and determines their optical treatment for abnormalities in their synkinetic near response. At this level, he soon comes to appreciate the clearer overall clinical picture that the distance-near measurements method affords. However, for most scientific investigations, the various controls that can be added to the lens gradient method, such as measuring accommodation response with the Badal optometer stigmatoscope (2) rather than depending on the accommodation stimulus and such as recording the accommodative convergence change with fixation disparity techniques (3) rather than with prism and alternate cover, make the lens gradient method the method of choice for the researcher studying the AC/A.

AMPLITUDE

Another parameter than can be used to assess accommodative convergence is its amplitude. The amplitude is a measure of the total prism diopter change in the alignment that is produced between totally relaxing the synkinetic near response and maximally applying it.

For example, an emmetropic child having a normal AC/A and an amplitude of accommodation of 14 diopters converges his eyes to a point 7 cm away when maximally accommodating. This quantity of convergence associated with the maximal accommodation is the maximal accommodative convergence. If the patient is orthophoric at dis-

tance and has an ideal AC/A, the amplitude of accommodative convergence equals the interpupillary distance in centimeters, times the amplitude of accommodation. Therefore, the amplitude of accommodative convergence usually ranges between 70Δ and 84Δ since the interpupillary distance of most children ranges from 5 to 6 cm. In contrast, a child with an amplitude of accommodation of 14D and a high AC/A that is relatively severe may have an amplitude of accommodative convergence of more than 150Δ. Another child with the same accommodation amplitude and a low AC/A may have an accommodative convergence amplitude of 40Δ or less.

Determining the amplitude of accommodation in any particular patient is not clinically helpful; its principal value is the concept it affords. As this discussion of the vergences continues, the fusional vergences will be evaluated entirely according to their amplitudes measured in prism diopters. Therefore, a method for relating accommodative convergence to the fusional vergence amplitude is important in order to appreciate all aspects of vergence; unfortunately, the AC/A does not supply this perspective. Once the amplitude of accommodative convergence is appreciated, one realizes that it is by far the strongest of all vergences.

FUSIONAL VERGENCE

Fusional vergence is an optomotor reflex. It produces corrective eye movements to overcome retinal image disparity. Fusional vergence is classified according to the plane of eye movements, ie, horizontal, vertical, or rotary. Horizontal fusional vergences are further subdivided into fusional convergence and divergence. Vertical fusional vergences are divided into positive and negative fusional vergence. Rotary fusional vergence is comprised of fusional incyclovergence and excyclovergence.

The maximal amount of eye movement produced by fusional vergence is referred to as an amplitude. The amplitudes of horizontal, vertical, and rotary fusional vergence are measurable; the prism diopter is the unit of measurement except in incyclovergence and excyclovergence, which are measured in degrees.

HORIZONTAL

Convergence

Fusional convergence is a reflex that responds only to the stimulus of bitemporal disparity of the retinal images. Since exotropia is associated with heteronymous diplopia resulting from the bitemporal image disparity, fusional convergence can overcome the diplopia by eliminating the retinal image disparity and maintaining exophoria.

The fusional convergence amplitude is measured by the maximal response to stimulation. The two clinical methods for stimulating fusional convergence are to adjust horizontal prism power before the eye or to converge the tubes of a major amblyoscope. Starting from the position of rest and evoking maximal fusional convergence with either the prisms or the major amblyoscope, the examiner determines the amplitude by directly reading the maximal response end-point. Accommodation must be controlled during the testing; otherwise, the patient could subconsciously apply the synkinetic near response to overcome the bitemporal disparity in retinal images. Accommodation is controlled by having the patient read small letters or numbers as his eyes converge; consequently, a muscle light and a small dot on a card do not qualify as accommodative targets. The examiner recognizes the maximal response end-point by noting the point at which the patient selects one of two options when the image disparity stimulus has just exceeded the fusional vergence amplitude. (1) The patient may apply the synkinetic near reflex in response to the image disparity that has just exceeded his fusional vergence amplitude; however, this is associated with accommodation, and since the accommodation is monitored with a detailed accommodative target, the patient reports blurring. (2) The patient may cease to further converge and may recognize diplopia; at that moment the examiner can see the patient's eyes break from the point of maximal convergence they achieved by the vergence reflex and drift to their resting position. This is called the fusion breakpoint. The examiner then reduces the retinal image disparity by reducing the prism power or the convergence of the major amblyoscope tubes until fusion is restored and the target is seen clearly. This is the fusion restoration point.

Either method requires that the examiner first know the status of the patient's refraction and compensate for it with corrective lenses so the accommodation is controlled. The patient is instructed in the end-points and told to report "blurring" or "doubling" as soon as it appears. The blurring is best illustrated to the patient by the examiner inserting +0.50 spheres before each eye while the patient views small letters at a distance of 6 meters. Similarly, the doubling is demonstrated by quickly inserting a 10Δ base-out prism before one of the patient's eyes and withdrawing it rapidly before the fusional response can be made.

The best prism technique for measuring the fusional convergence amplitude utilizes the rotary prism, which smoothly and slowly builds up the base-out prism power. Loose prisms or a horizontal prism bar may be used, but with each increment in prism power there is a momentary break in fusion and a restoration cycle that does not occur with the rotary prism. Although the test may be performed at any distance, 6 meters and 0.33 meter are customary. The fixation target at distance is a vision chart with numerous small letters; a small pocket calendar is a good target for near fixation.

The major amblyoscope may be used to measure the amplitude at either 6 meters or 0.33 meter. The near measurement is made by inserting -3.00 spheres in the oculus of each tube. The arms are steadily and slowly moved in from the objective setting until the end-point is reached. The slides in each housing are fusion slides (similar slides) with plenty of detail to control the accommodation.

The normal fusional convergence amplitude at 6 meters is 15Δ for fusion break and 12Δ for fusion restoration. This is usually recorded as 15/12. At 0.33 meter the amplitude normally is 20–25/18–22. The explanation for the near amplitude being invariably greater than the distant amplitude probably is related to the awareness of near and the awareness of far. At 6 meters the awareness of far dampens the use of the synkinetic near response to counter the bitemporal retinal image disparity that continues to build beyond the fusional convergence amplitude; however, at 0.33 meter the awareness of near encourages its use. Despite attempts to discourage the synkinetic near response by using techniques to control accommodation, some use of it escapes detection because of the depth of focus of the eye. The eye may be overaccommodated up to 1.50 D for the 0.33 meter target yet, due to the depth of focus, the vision is still clear. Therefore, it is very likely that the amplitude at 0.33 meter is a combination of fusional and accommodative convergence whereas the amplitude at 6 meters is a purer fusional convergence amplitude.

The above are the normal fusional convergence amplitudes found in orthophoria. Alignments that require fusional convergence to compensate for their deviation have larger amplitudes, while those who have no need for fusional convergence have smaller amplitudes; therefore, the amplitude is large in exophoria and small in esophoria. Orthoptic techniques have a great capability to effect a significant response in enlarging the amplitude and improving alignment control and symptoms in exophoria.

Divergence

Fusional divergence is a reflex that responds only to the stimulus of binasal retinal image disparity. The homonymous diplopia of esotropia caused by the binasal retinal image disparity can be overcome by fusional divergence, converting the strabismus to esophoria.

Fusional divergence amplitude is investigated by measuring its maximal response to stimulation. There are two direct methods and one indirect method for determining the fusional divergence amplitude. The two direct methods are the same as those described for measuring fusional convergence except that the horizontal prism power is increased in the opposite direction and the major amblyoscope tubes are diverged rather than converged. The necessity for controlling the accommodation and the end-points of response are the same as described in measuring fusional convergence.

The indirect method of measuring fusional divergence entails manipulating the synkinetic near response, increasing the binasal retinal image disparity by producing small increments of accommodative convergence until the amplitude of fusional divergence is just exceeded. The esotropia measured at this point by the prism and alternate cover test is equivalent to the fusional divergence amplitude. This can be performed at distance fixation or at near fixation; while the accommodation is controlled, minus-power lens increments are inserted in a trial frame before each eye. When diplopia with a sudden break of the eyes from fusion into overt estropia is produced, the lens increment has just exceeded the fusional divergence amplitude; the esotropia measured by prism and alternate cover through this lens is an indirect measure of the fusion breakpoint. The fusion restoration point is the esophoria measured through the weakest reduction in the lens power that allows fusional divergence to overcome the diplopia.

The normal fusional divergence amplitude at 6 meters is 8Δ for fusion break and 6Δ for fusion restoration. At 0.33 meter the amplitude normally is 12/9 and probably contains a small amount of accommodative convergence relaxation that is lacking in the amplitude at 6 meters. These are the usual and normal amplitudes encountered in orthophoria, but patients having esophoria tend to have larger fusional divergence amplitudes. Also, in the exophoric patient the amplitudes may be smaller than normal since there is no need for fusional divergence. The amplitude of fusional divergence may be expanded by orthoptic training, but it does not expand as easily nor to as great a degree as does the fusional convergence amplitude.

Relationship Between Horizontal Fusional Vergence and Synkinetic Near Reflex

Regardless of the method used to measure the amplitude of horizontal fusional vergence, attention must be given simultaneously to the synkinetic near reflex because it is an optomotor reflex that evokes a horizontal vergence. Since either reflex, ie, the horizontal fusional vergence or the synkinetic near reflex, is capable of overcoming horizontal disparity of retinal images, they must be differentiated from each other during investigation. Fusional convergence and accommodative convergence produce identical corrective eye movements, as do fusional divergence and relaxation of accommodative convergence. Therefore, a method that measures horizontal fusional vergence amplitude must eliminate the possibility of contamination of the results by accommodative convergence.

Fusional convergence and divergence are measured by two methods. In one method, accommodation is held constant while horizontal disparity of retinal images is produced by prisms or a haploscope. This method is called *relative convergence*. It is divided into two portions: (1) positive, which overcomes bitemporal retinal image disparity, and (2) negative, which overcomes binasal retinal image disparity. Positive relative convergence is fusional convergence and negative relative convergence is fusional divergence. In the other method, bifixation is maintained at a fixed distance while accommodation, and thus, accommodative convergence, is altered by plus and minus lenses. This method is called *relative accommodation*. Positive relative accommodation is produced by increasing accommodation, and negative relative accommodation is produced by decreasing accommodation. To maintain bifixation, positive relative accommodation requires fusional divergence and negative relative accommodation requires fusional convergence. If prism and alternate cover measurements are made first while maintaining maximal positive relative accommodation and secondly while maintaining maximal negative relative accommodation, the findings are equivalent to the fusional divergence and convergence amplitudes, respectively. Therefore, the examiner may employ either the technique of positive relative convergence or that of negative relative accommodation to measure the amplitude of the fusional convergence. Similarly, either the technique of negative relative convergence or that of positive relative accommodation may be used to measure the amplitude of the fusional divergence.

VERTICAL

Positive

Positive vertical vergence is a simultaneous elevation of the right eye and depression of the left eye, compensating for a left hyperdeviation by maintaining a left hyperphoria.

Negative

Negative vertical vergence is the opposite of positive vertical vergence, viz, maintaining right hyperphoria by simultaneous depression of the right eye and elevation of the left eye.

Vertical fusional vergence amplitudes are measured by producing vertical retinal image disparity with prisms or the major amblyoscope. To stimulate positive vertical vergence, either the image on the right retina is lowered or the image on the left retina is raised by increasing base-down prism power before the right eye or base-up prism power before the left eye. Stimulation of negative vertical fusion requires the opposite. The major amblyoscope accomplishes the same results by appropriately moving the tubes vertically in opposite directions before the right and the left eye. Directing the tube before the right eye downward and the tube before the left eye upward measures positive vertical fusional vergence; moving the tubes in opposite direction measures negative fusional vergence.

Accommodation does not have to be controlled during measurement of vertical vergence amplitude, since the synkinetic near reflex cannot influence the findings. The end-point of the fusional vergence amplitude is diplopia. A normal amplitude is 3Δ to 6Δ, depending on how slowly the measurement is made. Left hyperphoria patients have a greater positive than negative vertical vergence amplitude, whereas the reverse is true in patients having right hyperphoria.

TORSIONAL

Incyclovergence is simultaneous incycloduction of each eye to compensate for exocyclodeviation and to maintain excyclophoria.

Excyclovergence is simultaneous excycloduction of each eye to compensate for incyclodeviation and to maintain incyclophoria.

The amplitude of torsional fusional vergences is measured on the major amblyoscope by rotating the housings in which the slides are placed until cyclodiplopia is produced. The only end-point of the torsional vergence amplitude is cyclodiplopia. The normal patient has an incyclovergence of 6° to 10° and an excyclovergence of 8° to 12°.

TONIC VERGENCES

The innervational factor that produces a vergence movement that is neither a fusional vergence nor an accommodative convergence is designated tonic. Tonic vergences are most commonly referred to as having a horizontal plane of action and are divided into tonic convergence and divergence. The tonic vergences defy measurement, so there is no known way to investigate them. Presumably tonic convergence and divergence check one another and account for the near orthophoria encountered in most patients who are not accommodating and in whom fusion is precluded by the alternate cover test. A disturbance in the balance of tonic convergence and divergence is the usual explanation for certain horizontal tropias. For example, congenital esotropia is thought to result if an infant has an excess of tonic convergence or a deficiency of tonic divergence; exotropia results from the reverse. There is some merit in this simple concept since both tropias reduce toward orthophoria when the patient is under anesthesia providing there is no peripheral mechanical factor restricting passive adduction or abduction. Also, an increase in tonic convergence is thought to account for the increasing esodeviation associated with fatigue, illness, and emotional disturbances. The fact that straight eyes become increasingly esophoric for distance fixation as the alcohol level in the blood increases or with progressive anoxemia is explained by such toxic factors stimulating tonic convergence.

REFERENCES

1. Duane A: A new classification of the anomalies of the eye, based upon physiological principles. Ann Ophthalmol Part I, October 1896, Part II, January 1897
2. Alpern M: Vergence and accommodation. Arch Ophthalmol 60:358, 1958
3. Ogle KN: On the accommodative covergence and the proximal convergence. Arch Ophthalmol 57:702, 1957

8

Sensorial Adaptations in Strabismus

Infants and children having congenital strabismus have no untoward visual sensations. Their only visual handicap is absence of stereopsis, but they no more are able to comprehend this deficiency than those who are color-blind are able to comprehend their deficiency in color perception.

BINOCULAR VISION

Cortical integration of similar images on each retina into a unified perception is single binocular vision. Once established, binocular vision is retained as long as there is sight in both eyes. One cannot escape this reflex even though it may prove troublesome. If the benefits of single binocular vision are lost due to distruption in the alignment or due to the optical state of the eyes, binocular vision annoyingly continues in the form of diplopia and visual confusion. Fortunately, young children can adapt their binocular vision to the misalignment or the disturbed optical state, thus solving the annoying binocular vision by such ingenious compensatory cortical adjustments as suppression and anomalous retinal correspondence (ARC).

SYMPTOMS OF STRABISMUS

If single binocular vision has developed, symptoms will appear as soon as strabismic eyes deviate.

Diplopia

Diplopia is the simultaneous perception of two images of one object resulting from these similar images projecting onto noncorresponding retinal areas. The simultaneous perception of images under these circumstances yields the impression that the object of regard is simultaneously located at two points in space (Fig 8-1). If the deviation is sufficiently small to displace only objects in the area of conscious regard onto noncorresponding retinal areas, peripheral objects still project onto corresponding retinal areas (Fig 8-2). Diplopia extends to *all* objects in visual space when their images are projected onto noncorresponding retinal areas; therefore, simultaneously there is diplopia for both the area of conscious regard (central diplopia) and the peripheral vision (peripheral diplopia).

Visual Confusion

Visual confusion results when dissimilar images, normally projected onto noncorresponding retinal areas, project onto corresponding retinal areas, as occurs in strabismus. Consequently, these different

Not all patients with strabismus adapt their binocular vision to conform to the deviation of their eyes; this facility apparently is confined to the young. Also, some strabismic patients have no binocular vision, and therefore no adaptation is possible.

ABSENCE OF BINOCULAR VISION

Binocular vision is an acquired physiologic reflex that develops during the first several months of life. Its development demands certain requisites. Each eye must be capable of seeing, and both eyes must be aligned within the first few years of life to permit the projection of similar images onto corresponding retinal areas. The latter requisite is lacking in patients with congenital strabismus. Their misaligned eyes never receive similar images on corresponding retinal areas; consequently, binocular vision is not developed. Absence of binocular vision is made manifest by sensory tests yielding responses that prove the absence of simultaneous perception of images on each retina. Despite the absence of simultaneous perception, attention directed to the area of conscious regard first with one eye and then with the other results in alternate fixation of the object. If attention to the area of conscious regard is exclusively with one eye, this monocular fixation habit results in amblyopia of the unused eye.

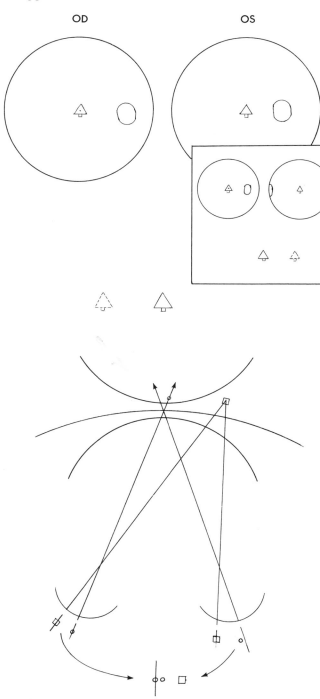

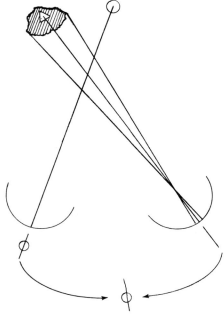

Fig 8-1. Diplopia results from simultaneous perception of similar images projecting onto noncorresponding retinal areas. Esotropia causes homonymous diplopia; clear image on macula of right eye is illustrated by solid lines, blurred image on nasal retina of left eye is illustrated by broken lines. The illustrated diplopic images are according to the patient's drawing of them. **Insert.** Heteronymous diplopia in exotropia.

Fig 8-3. An absolute physiologic scotoma projects into space from the macular area of the deviated eye immediately when the eye deviates, preventing perception simultaneously of an image on the deviated macula that is dissimilar to the macular image of the fixating eye.

Fig 8-2. The heterotropic deviation may be sufficiently small to cause the object of regard to be diplopic, but the peripheral objects displaced equidistant to the object of regard from the horopter may still be within Panum's area. Thus, it is possible for a patient with a small heterotropic deviation to have peripheral fusion in the absence of central fusion.

objects in space creating dissimilar images are perceived as located at the same place in space. Visual confusion does not exist for all portions of the visual field. The object of regard is not superimposed by a different object projecting on the fovea of the deviating eye (Fig 8-3). This is due to the physiologic fact of binocular vision that only similar images on the rod-free retinal areas are perceived simultaneously; no binocular function results from the dissimilar images on these retinal areas. Consequently, from the moment the strabismic eyes deviate the patient is spared visual confusion for the object of regard. An absolute scotoma of the macula of the deviated eye can be plotted using a binocular perimetric technique, but this is a physiologic scotoma, present in all age-groups immediately on onset of strabismus—not a pathologic scotoma that can only evolve gradually in a child to resolve an annoying visual symptom.

ADAPTATIONS TO STRABISMUS

Physical Adaptations

The onset of strabismus in a person who has developed single binocular vision produces three distinct, annoying symptoms: central diplopia, peripheral diplopia, and peripheral visual confusion. Two factors offer partial relief from central diplopia. One is the perceptual difference in the sharpness and clearness of the two similar images since one is projected onto the fovea and the other onto an extramacular area. This difference, however, pertains only to visual stimuli with contour value that are viewed during the photopic state. To compensate for this visual circumstance, important clues are provided for the strabismic patient to locate the object of regard correctly in space. However, when using scotopic vision or when viewing a contourless object such as a light, the patient does not have these differential clues of sharpness and clearness for the object of regard; consequently, the diplopia persists unabated.

Secondly, the ability to be attentive to only one of the images of the object of regard is subconsciously enhanced by a rapid blinking of the nondominant eye. The image that correctly localizes the object of regard is immediately identified, and as long as the patient's attention remains attached to this image, correct localization of the object continues. This functions satisfactorily as long as the object of regard remains unchanging, but with scotopia, if the patient is viewing a series of changing contourless objects such as multiple oncoming headlights during nighttime driving, only sustained voluntary closure of the nondominant eye may avert catastrophe.

Cortical Adaptations

Eventual relief from the troublesome symptoms of central and peripheral diplopia and peripheral visual confusion is obtained for some patients through cortical adaptations that occur within the neurophysiology of single binocular vision. Development of these complex adaptations is limited to the very young strabismic patient; children over 10 years of age are incapable of acquiring them. As already mentioned, once binocular vision is acquired, it is never surrendered. Also, once single binocular vision has developed, the strabismic patient attempts to maintain it; however, only the young patient successfully de-

velops suppression and ARC, the adaptations necessary to permit continuation of single binocular vision. Older patients are permanent victims of the annoying symptoms caused by their continuing binocular vision.

SUPPRESSION. Suppression is a positive inhibitory reflex occurring within the framework of binocular vision; it permits the cortex to ignore visual sensations dispatched from the retina of the nonfixating eye upon which are projected the images from the area of conscious regard. This adaptation eliminates central diplopia. If either eye can maintain fixation, suppression is demonstrable in each nonfixating eye. In contrast to the physiologic macular scotoma that can be plotted in the deviated eye, the extramacular suppression scotoma is pathologic. It is absolute, but it is also facultative since it is nonexistent during monocular vision. Therefore, it may be plotted only during binocular perimetry. The shape and the size of the suppression scotoma in esotropia (Fig 8-4) differ significantly from the scotoma in exotropia. The nasal retina in esotropia usually has a scotoma of approximately 5°, while the temporal retina in exotropia produces a scotoma extending peripheralward from the hemiretinal line for the number of degrees required to extinguish the image of the object of regard. This difference in size of the scotomas probably relates to the intermittence of strabismus during the forma-

Fig 8-4. The scotoma in an extropic patient extensively involves temporal retina up to the hemiretinal line; in the nasal retina of the esotropic patient **(Insert),** it is small and regional.

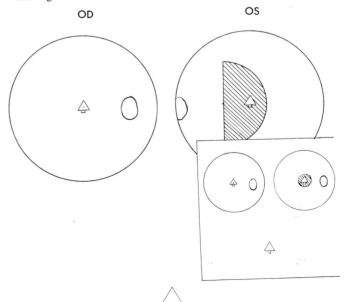

tive period of the suppression. Esotropia usually is more constant compared to the intermittence of exotropia. Consequently, in esotropia the image of the object of regard is almost constantly directed to one small region of the nasal retina, but in intermittent exotropia it sweeps frequently across a temporal region of the retina equivalent to the angle of the deviation, as tropia and phoria vie with one another.

ARC. Anomalous retinal correspondence is the cortical adjustment in directional values supplied by the neuroepithelial retinal elements for strabismic eyes to permit fusion of the similar images projected onto noncorresponding areas by object points peripheral to the area of conscious regard. Anomalous retinal correspondence is the adaptation that eliminates peripheral diplopia and peripheral visual confusion in strabismus. Patients with vertical strabismus and those with horizontal strabismus develop ARC to eliminate diplopia and visual confusion.

No matter which eye fixates—whether there is foveal fixation in both eyes or eccentric fixation in one eye—ARC is present. It is manifest only during binocular seeing; there is no abnormality in the directional values of the neuroepithelial elements of either eye during monocular seeing.

Once ARC has developed and peripheral single binocular vision is present in the strabismic patient, he is always able to cortically adjust the directional values supplied by the neuroepithelial retinal elements to permit continuous fusion of similar images, in spite of different positions the eyes may assume. Subsequent to any change of eye alignment, such as after surgery, an ARC patient experiences diplopia and visual confusion until cortical adjustment is adapted to match the directional values of the retinal neuroepithelial elements to the new alignment. This reflex conditioning requires time, often several week for adults but usually only a few days for children, but the cortical adjustment is finally reconciled.

There is no apparent reason why ARC should not be a total cortical adjustment of the directional values of the retinal neuroepithelial elements to the degree that would allow fusion. Yet, the results of certain testing techniques that do not simulate everyday seeing experience suggest that only a partial cortical adjustment occurs in some patients. From these results, the classifications of harmonious ARC and unharmonious ARC have evolved to describe total and partial cortical adjustment. The results of recent nonlaboratory testing, offering

everyday seeing experiences, indicate that the unharmonious ARC response is an artifact produced by the artificial seeing circumstance in the retinal correspondence test. The classic test for ARC with the major amblyoscope evokes these artifactual responses.

The ability of peripheral single binocular vision to provide good fusional vergence amplitudes has been discussed previously. Although ARC is peripheral fusion in a strabismic setting, evidence does not support the existence of fusional vergence amplitudes associated with this cortically adjusted peripheral fusion. Any fusional vergence amplitudes possessed by ARC patients are extremely limited. This may be explained by the fact that ARC patients have no need for fusional vergence amplitudes. It is more reasonable to expect the ARC patient to make a cortical adaptation in the visual direction of the retinal neuroepithelial elements to conform with the eye alignment than to expect him to make a motor response to alter the alignment in behalf of fusion. Therefore, ARC is a sensory peripheral fusion adaptation without a motor component, unlike fusion in normal retinal correspondence (NRC), which possesses both a sensory and a motor component.

Another deficiency encountered in ARC patients involves stereopsis. There was no stereopsis appreciation in ARC patients who had a simultaneous prism and cover deviation greater than 8Δ when tested with Polaroid vectographic targets that created a retinal image disparity of 6,000 seconds of arc (using the Polaroid vectographic housefly of the Titmus Stereotest (Fig 8-5) held 20 cm from the eyes).

Anomalous retinal correspondence and suppression (Fig 8-6) seem to develop simultaneously in most patients. With various testing techniques, they are easily demonstrated coexisting in the esotrope; however, this is usually not so easily demonstrated in the exotrope. The suppression scotoma in the deviated eye of the esotrope is small and confined to a retinal area of 5°, and the retinal area surrounding it is readily tested. This contrasts to the profound suppression scotoma of the temporal retina in the deviated eye of the exotrope; it extends up to the hemiretinal line which may measure 20° or more, making it difficult for the patient to observe images projected on the retina peripheral to the scotomatous region (Fig 8-4).

Patients with intermittent strabismus may have ARC and suppression while the eyes are deviated but NRC and no suppression when the eyes are straight. Also, patients having deviation angles

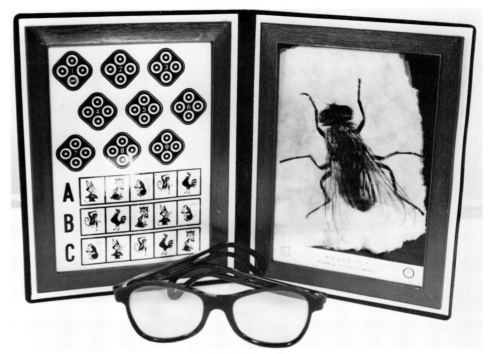

Fig 8-5. Titmus Stereotest.

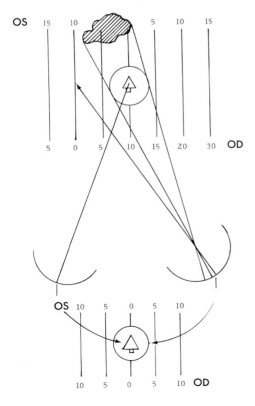

Fig 8-6. Anomalous retinal correspondence is the cortical adjustment in strabismus that permits fusion of similar images projecting onto noncorresponding retinal areas from object points peripheral to the area of conscious regard. Suppression eliminates the diplopia caused by object points within the area of conscious regard projecting onto noncorresponding retinal areas.

that vary in different positions of gaze may have ARC values and suppression scotoma localization that change according to the deviation angle as the eyes are moved into various positions; this is commonly seen in strabismic patients whose horizontal deviation has an associated A or V pattern. Lastly, some patients with double hyperdeviations may have single binocular vision that vacillates, with either eye intermittently elevating. While the eyes are on the same level, single binocular vision prevails, but as one or the other dissociates and drifts upward, single binocular vision is immediately lost. The cortical integrating mechanism for the similar retinal images is very supple and elastic in some tropia patients and totally inelastic and rigid in others. The former is encountered in patients having variable strabismus during infancy and early childhood, and the latter is encountered in those who first manifest their strabismus in later childhood or as adults.

Young esotropic patients having 25Δ to 40Δ of deviation may use the blind spot of the deviated eye as the suppression scotoma (Fig 8-7), removing the need for their cortex to adapt to the central diplopia. However, their retinal area peripheral to the blind spot may adapt to the peripheral diplopia and develop ARC. Such a patient has no cortical adaptation equivalent to suppression but does have the cortical adaptation of ARC, an example of a situation in which both cortical adaptations do not develop concomitantly.

Consequently, one cannot state that suppression and ARC invariably are associated cortical adaptations of the normal single binocular vision.

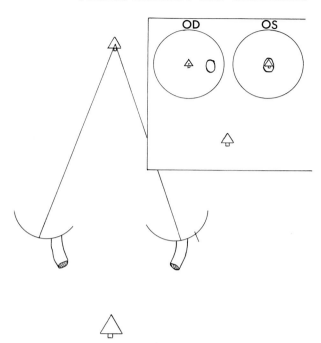

Fig 8-7. The physiologic blind spot offers an excellent immediate scotoma for the esotropic patient having 25Δ to 35Δ of deviation.

9

Sensory Tests

WORTH 4 DOT TEST

One of the simpler tests for fusion, suppression, and anomalous retinal correspondence (ARC) is the Worth 4 dot, which can be done at any distance from the patient. The patient, wearing a red filter before one eye and a green filter before the other, is exposed to four lights: two green, one red, and one white. In normal individuals, the white light is seen through both filters, the green lights are seen only through the green filter, and the red light is seen only through the red filter. The patient with fusion reports that there are four lights, but the white light is a mixture of red and green, ever changing due to color rivalry. The test is performed with ordinary room illumination to provide the usual peripheral vision clues.

The projection angle of the dots may be increased or decreased many degrees, either by having the patient approach or move away from the distant Worth dots or by moving the near Worth dots nearer to or farther from the patient. At 6 meters the distant Worth dots project an image of 1.25°, and at 0.33 meter the near Worth dots project a 6° angle (Fig 9-1). The projection angle of the image is the imaginary circumference encircling the outer border of the four dots collectively, not simply the projection angle of each of the four dots. Since the macular area is approximately 3°, the dots can be a test for bimacular fusion (central fusion) or extramacular fusion (peripheral fusion), depending on the projection angle of the dots offered to the patient. A person fusing the distant Worth 4 dots at 6 meters has

central fusion. The patient should be tested with whatever optical correction is required to provide good monocular acuity in each eye, particularly if a small projection angle is presented to the patient.

Some patients with straight eyes and certainly those having a horizontal deviation no larger than 8Δ of straight by the simultaneous prism and cover test may suppress the Worth 4 dots only when their projection angle is less than 3° because of a macular scotoma that is always present in the nonfixating eye. The suppression response is manifest by the patient seeing either three green or two red dots; these may alternate if he switches fixation from one eye to the other. The peripheral fusion in these patients is apparent by their fusion response for larger projection angles of the Worth 4 dots (Fig 9-2).

Patients with esotropia of 10Δ or greater will not fuse the distant Worth 4 dots. Normal retinal correspondence (NRC) is identified by the response that five lights (two red and three green) are seen. The dots seen by the fixating eye are clear, whereas those seen by the deviating eye are blurred. The red and green dots are homonymously projected, and fusion may be produced when the deviation angle is corrected with base-out prisms equal to the deviation angle. Anomalous retinal correspondence is obscured by the suppression response of the deviated eye until the projection angle of the Worth dots exceeds 5° to 6°, at which time the ARC fusion response becomes apparent (Fig 9-3). When the projection angle is increased sufficiently so all dots are imaged outside the nasal scotoma, the fusion response is not accompanied by color rivalry of the white dot. Instead, the white dot remains the sustained color of the filter before the fixating eye. Placing base-out prisms equal to the esotropia angle before the eyes converts the fusion response to crossed diplopia of the red and green dots. An absence of single binocular vision is seen when the patient never fuses the Worth dots, regardless of how closely he approaches the distant dots or how close the near dots are brought to the eyes (Fig 9-4). The patient continues to see either three green or two red dots even though his face is 15 cm away from the distant Worth 4 dots or the near Worth 4 dots are only 7 cm from his eyes.

The exotropic patient may not respond similarly to the esotropic patient because of the large temporal suppression scotoma extending up to the hemiretinal line. If this large scotoma is present, ARC may not be evident until the angle of deviation is compensated for by placing the full correction of a base-in prism equal to the strabismic angle before

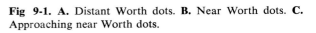

Fig 9-1. **A.** Distant Worth dots. **B.** Near Worth dots. **C.** Approaching near Worth dots.

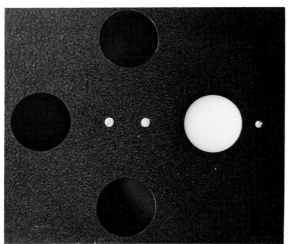

A

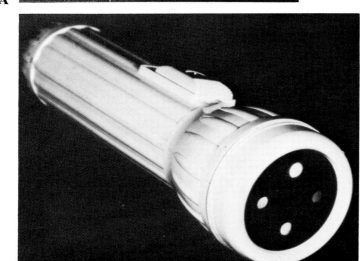

B

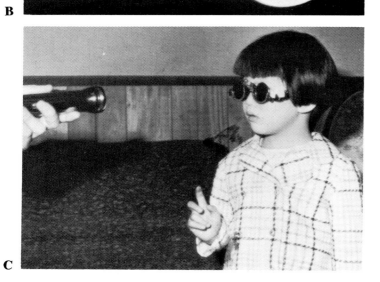

C

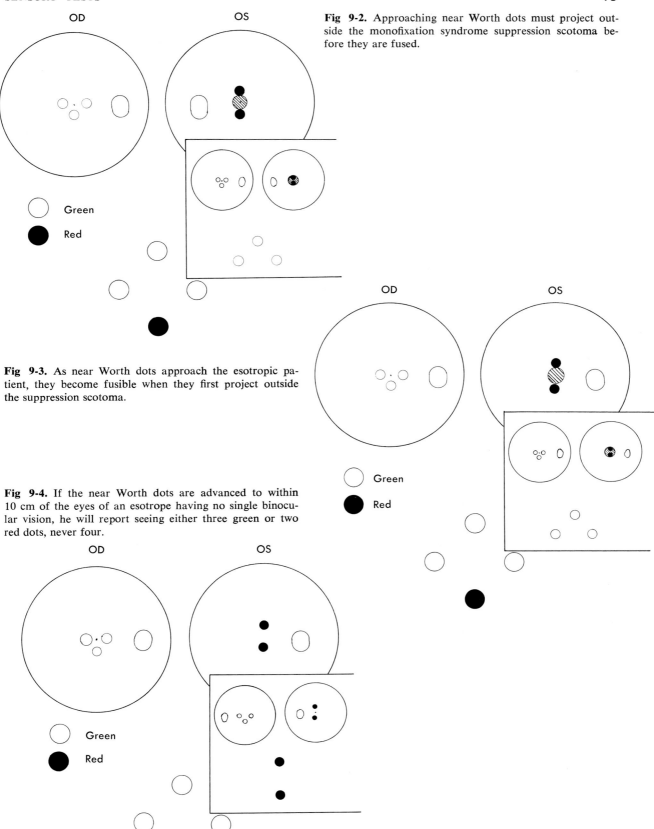

OD   OS

Fig 9-2. Approaching near Worth dots must project outside the monofixation syndrome suppression scotoma before they are fused.

Green

Red

Fig 9-3. As near Worth dots approach the esotropic patient, they become fusible when they first project outside the suppression scotoma.

Fig 9-4. If the near Worth dots are advanced to within 10 cm of the eyes of an esotrope having no single binocular vision, he will report seeing either three green or two red dots, never four.

OD   OS

Green

Red

OD   OS

Green

Red

the eyes, producing homonymous diplopia for the red and green dots.

The Worth 4 dot test is simple enough to be performed on children who can count to five. Usually, if the visual acuity can be determined, so also can the Worth 4 dot response. One precaution must be exercised in performing the test on strabismic children. Occasionally the child will rapidly switch fixation; he will have no single binocular vision and yet will report five lights by simply adding the two and the three response. The examiner must determine whether the five lights are seen simultaneously or if they are the summation of the separate three-two responses.

BAGOLINI STRIATED GLASSES TEST

Most tests for fusion, suppression, and ARC create artificial viewing circumstances. Normally the visual environment is not viewed through a red filter before one eye or through a combination of red-green filters; separately viewed slides in illuminated tubes are nothing more than a laboratory analysis of retinal correspondence. However, the striated glasses popularized by Bagolini (Fig 9-5) allow the patient to view the normal visual environment with a faint reference line placed on the background viewed by each eye. The reference line for each eye is placed at right angles by arranging the glasses

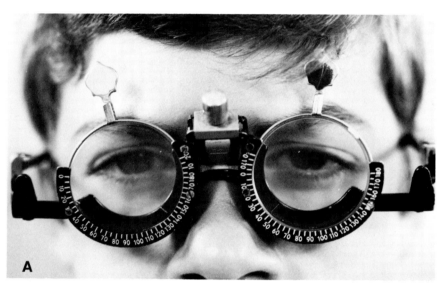

A

OD   OS

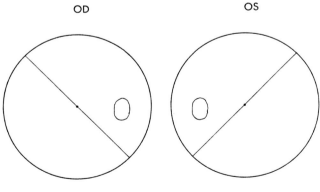

B

Fig 9-5. A. Bagolini striated glasses. **B.** Simultaneous perception of opposite diagonal streaks projected onto opposite retinas by Bagolini striated glasses in person without strabismus.

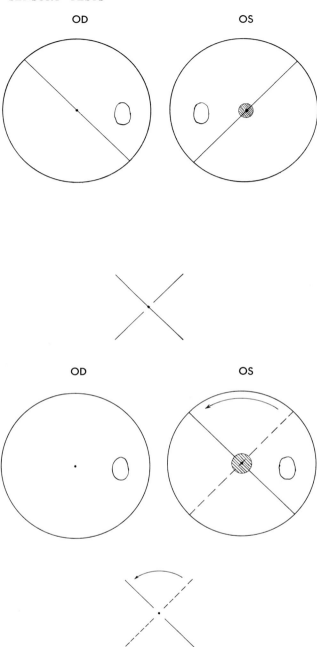

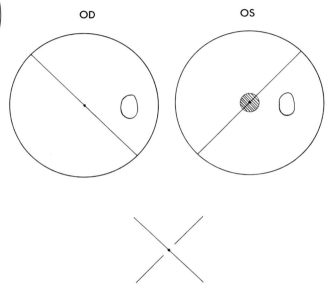

Fig 9-6. Monofixation syndrome with left eye suppression manifested by Bagolini striated glasses.

Fig 9-7. Esotropic patient having ARC and suppression elicits single binocular vision adaptations simultaneously with the Bagolini striated glasses test.

OD   OS

OD   OS

Fig 9-8. Scotoma in deviated esotropic eye can be outlined with the Bagolini striated glasses.

in the trial frame so that the striations before the right eye and the left eye are perpendicular to one another. For example, the striations are placed at 135° in the trial frame before the right eye and at 45° before the left eye. The subject views a fixation light at any distance the examiner chooses; ordinary room illumination is maintained. The subject re-

ports on the fixation light and observed streaks extending out into the peripheral field of vision.

Patients with either straight eyes or with a deviation up to 8Δ by simultaneous prism and cover test and NRC single binocular vision describe seeing one fixation light and two streaks forming an **X** intersecting at the light. The bifixating patient with central fusion sees it as just described. If central fusion is lacking although peripheral fusion is present, a gap of 3° is reported in one streak on either side of the light (Fig 9-6). The gap represents the macular scotoma in the nonfixating eye of the monofixating patient. Monofixating patients are unaware of this gap in the one streak around the fixating light until the examiner questions them about it; they invariably seem to be oblivious to the presence of the scotoma until it is brought to their attention. When the fixating eye is covered, the gap in the streak disappears, and the entire streak then passes through the center of the fixation light. If the patient can switch fixation, the macular scotoma is observed to transfer from eye to eye.

Patients with esotropia of 10Δ or greater give varied responses depending on whether they have NRC or ARC single binocular vision or an absence of single binocular vision. The NRC esotropic patient sees two fixation lights in homonymous diplopia with a separate streak·through each and

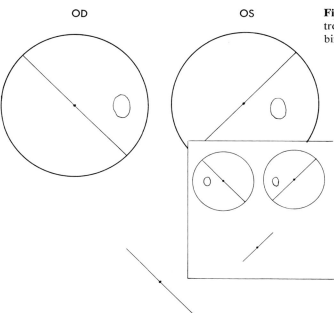

Fig 9-9. Response to Bagolini striated glasses in an eso-trope having alternating fixation and absence of single binocular vision.

without a break in either streak. Compensating for the esotropic angle with base-out prisms eliminates the diplopic fixation light, and the streaks then intersect at the fixation light. The patient with ARC and suppression sees one fixation light and two streaks forming an X; after questioning he recognizes the suppression scotoma projecting from the nasal retina of the deviated eye as a gap of 5° to 6° around the fixation light in the streak seen by that eye (Fig 9-7). The scotoma can be further studied by removing the striated glass from in front of the fixating eye and then slowly rotating the striated glass before the nonfixating eye (Fig 9-8). As the streak rotates, the gap in the streak around the fixation light persists, beautifully outlining the scotoma for 360°. Furthermore, the ARC is made evident by the patient's claim that the streak seen by the deviated eye passes through the fixation light as he mentally connects the two ends of the gap in this streak. When held before the eyes, base-out prism power equal to the esotropic deviation produces crossed diplopia for the fixation light, and each light has its separate streak passing through it. The patient devoid of single binocular vision sees only one light and one streak (Fig 9-9). He may claim to see two streaks if he rapidly alternates, but he will admit under questioning that they are not perceived simultaneously.

The patient with exotropia of 10Δ or more may report NRC with heteronymous diplopia, ARC with suppression, or an absence of single binocular vision. The large profound scotoma of the temporal retina, extending up to the hemiretinal line

Fig 9-10. The large suppression scotoma in an exotropic patient often causes the Bagolini striated glasses stimulus in the deviated eye to remain unrecognized.

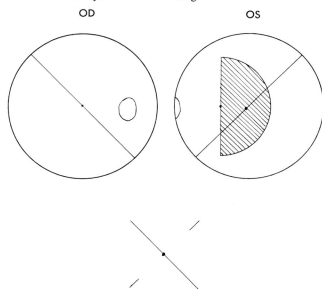

in the exotropic patient with ARC, prevents all but the best observers from appreciating the extremely peripheral, small streak seen outside the suppression scotoma of the deviated eye (Fig 9-10); consequently, many exotropic patients report seeing only one streak. Those who can detect the small peripheral ends of the streak describe the ends on the axis that coincides with the light, supporting the diagnosis of ARC. Furthermore, base-in prism power placed before the eyes that equals the deviation angle creates homonymous diplopia of the fixation light, each image having a separate streak.

The Bagolini striated lens test requires a degree of maturity that is seldom found in a child under 8 years of age. Describing or drawing the suppression scotoma gap in one of the streaks presents great difficulty to the young child.

MAJOR AMBLYOSCOPE TEST

Fusion is investigated with the major amblyoscope by placing appropriate fusion targets (Fig 5-7, *B*) in the housing of each tube and adjusting the instrument to project the similar images onto corresponding retinal areas of each eye. The fusion targets are identical except for one detail. For example, the target may be a clown identical in every detail on the right and left slides except that the hat is lacking from the right slide and the cane from the left. The report that the clown has both the hat and the cane indicates fusion. It is a great advantage that the tubes of this instrument can be adjusted according to the strabismus angle, enabling the targets to project onto corresponding retinal areas.

After the presence of sensory fusion has been ascertained with this instrument, further testing is natural to investigate the motor aspect of fusion by determining the fusional vergence amplitudes. The technique for this determination is described in the chapter titled Vergences.

Retinal correspondence in a strabismic patient is also investigated on the major amblyoscope. For this test the targets must be dissimilar, eg, a fish and a bowl (Fig 5-7, *A*). If the patient has single binocular vision he will simultaneously perceive the dissimilar images projected on each retina. The tubes are set at the objective angle (the adjustment that compensates for all refixation movements of the eyes as the tubes are alternately illuminated while the center of each target is alternately fixated), which measures the angle of the strabismus. Next, the patient is asked to adjust the tubes so that the targets appear superimposed; this reveals the subjective angle. Objective and subjective angles that are identical indicate NRC; those that are dissimilar indicate ARC. A subjective setting of zero by a strabismic patient is harmonious ARC, indicating that the cortical adaptation of ARC fully compensates for the angle of strabismus. A subjective angle that is somewhere between zero and the objective angle is unharmonious ARC, indicating that the cortical adaptation of ARC does

not fully compensate for the angle of strabismus. Actually, the ARC patient usually experiences some difficulty in superimposing the targets at the subjective angle, eg, as he approaches the lion toward one end of the cage it suddenly disappears, only to reappear as it leaves the other end of the cage, due to the suppression scotoma coexisting with ARC.

RED FILTER TEST

Fusion is tested by viewing a muscle light with both eyes while a red filter is maintained before one eye (Fig 6-10). A nondiplopic response and an appreciation of a pink light suggests central fusion. Individually, one eye views the light as white while the other views it as red, but in accordance with the laws of color fusion, the fused perception is a pink tint.

Suppression is tested by placing the red filter before the nondominant eye. A report that only the white light is seen suggests that the red image is projecting within the suppression scotoma. The alignment of the eyes determines the retinal locus from which the scotoma projects. In patients with straight eyes or in those whose deviation by simultaneous prism and cover is 8Δ or less, the scotoma includes the macula; in strabismic patients with greater deviations, the scotoma projects from an extramacular region.

The size and profoundness of the scotoma is investigated next. As previously discussed in the chapter titled Sensorial Adaptations to Strabismus, the nasal scotoma in esotropia is approximately 5° to 6°, while the temporal scotoma in exotropia is usually much larger and extends up to the hemiretinal line. The depth of the scotoma may vary from slight to profound. Rapidly covering and uncovering the eye with minimal suppression for just a few moments may be sufficient to produce appreciation of diplopia. If suppression persists despite flashing of the occluder, the examiner introduces a 15Δ base-up or base-down prism before the red filter. This is usually sufficient (in esotropes at least) to move the red image out of the suppression area. If diplopia still is not reported, the examiner wiggles the prism in a rocking manner; this constantly moves the image on the retina. If many attempts with the latter technique are required to awake diplopia, the suppression scotoma is indeed profound. In many exotropes, the scotoma is so profound that diplopia is never recognized by the patient.

Once diplopia can be maintained, the examiner can proceed with an analysis of the retinal correspondence, even if a 15Δ base-down prism must be held constantly before the eye behind the red filter. First, the horizontal nature of the diplopia must be established. The absence of any horizontal displacement when there is a horizontal strabismus, regardless of whether it is esotropia or exotropia, is diagnostic of harmonious ARC. Horizontal displacement of the lights, which is homonymous for esotropia and heteronymous for exotropia, indicates there is either NRC or unharmonious ARC. To differentiate, base-out prism power for esotropia and base-in power for exotropia is introduced until the white and red lights are seen without horizontal separation. A convenient method for introducing this prism power is to use either the horizontal prism bar or the rotary prism. If the strabismus angle and the prism power required to vertically align the diplopic images are approximately the same, the patient has NRC; otherwise, he has unharmonious ARC.

LANCASTER PROJECTORS

Another method of investigating the retinal correspondence in a strabismic patient entails use of the Lancaster red-green projectors (Fig 6-11). The red-green filters used in the Worth 4 dot test are worn by the patient. One projector shines a red target and the other a green target on a calibrated screen 1 meter from the patient. The patient controls the adjustment of the projectors; while keeping one on zero (screen center), he is to arrange the targets so they become superimposed (subjective angle). The calibrated screen offers the examiner a direct reading of the subjective angle of the patient. If the examiner already knows the objective angle from prism and alternate cover testing, a comparison is readily made between the objective and the subjective angle. The two angles are equal in NRC and dissimilar in ARC. Superimposition of both the red and the green target on zero indicates that the ARC is harmonious. Superimposition of the targets at an angle between the angle of strabismus and zero indicates unharmonious ARC.

AFTERIMAGE TEST

The retinal correspondence in older strabismic children who have central fixation ability in each eye may be investigated with the afterimage test. A linear electric filament approximately 30 cm long is the basic component of the instrument. An area approximately 4 cm long in the center of the filament is blocked out so that when the filament is turned on, it appears as two illuminated filaments 13 cm long, separated by a 4-cm nonilluminated gap. The patient's attention is directed to a fixation spot in the center of the gap. The illuminated filament is offered vertically for approximately 15 seconds to the right eye while the left eye is shielded and then horizontally for the same time to the left eye while the right is covered (Fig 9-11). This technique produces vertical and horizontal afterimages, each having a central gap. Positive afterimages are seen with either eye closed or in the dark, while negative afterimages are experienced with the eyes open in an illuminated room. Negative afterimages are best brought out by intermittent illumination, ie, by flickering the lights off and on, since these images tend to wash out rapidly in sustained illumination. A report from the patient that the afterimages form a cross signifies NRC. A vertical afterimage line that is displaced away from the break in the horizontal afterimage line is found in ARC. In esotropia with ARC, the afterimages are heteronymous; the image seen by the right eye is left and that by the left eye is right. The images are homonymous in exotropia with ARC. Occasionally a patient with tropia reports NRC with positive afterimages and ARC with negative afterimages. This peculiar finding means that the patient uses the innate NRC system when his eyes are not exposed to clues in the environment but he shifts to the adapted ARC system when his eyes are in the open. The implication of this finding is that the prognosis is better for a return to fusion with NRC after the squint angle has been eliminated than the prognosis in the case in which ARC is present with both positive and negative afterimages.

4△ BASE-OUT TEST

The 4△ base-out test is useful in patients whose eyes appear straight to determine whether bifixation (central fusion) or monofixation (absence of central fusion) exists. While the patient reads letters at a distance of 6 meters, a 4△ base-out prism is slipped before first one eye and then the other. The prism-covered eye is watched closely for movement.

Fig 9-11. Afterimage test. **A.** Vertical filament stimulation. **B.** Horizontal filament stimulation.

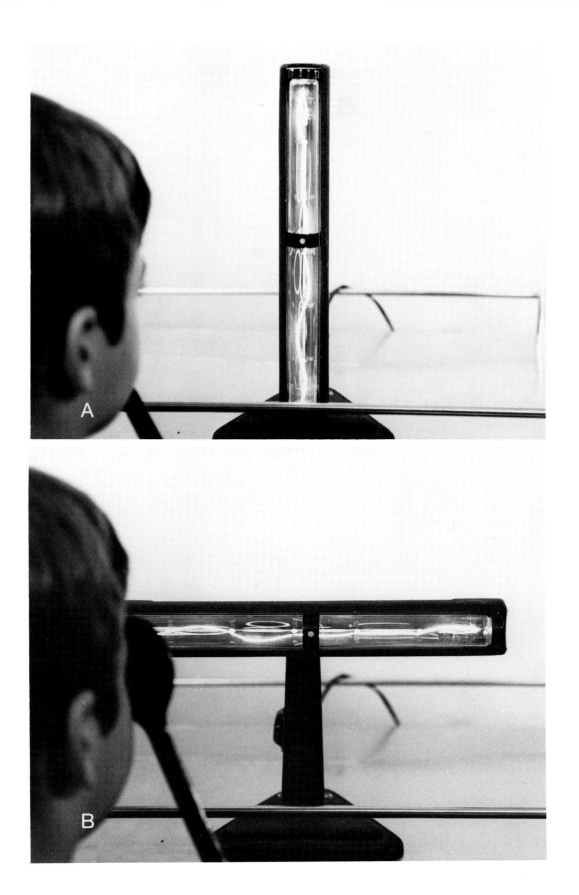

A

B

Absence of movement by one of the eyes is proof of a macular scotoma in that eye. Bifixation is identified by each eye moving inward to refixate in response to the image displacement produced by the prism. The test is not completely reliable since occasionally bifixating patients recognize diplopia when the prism is slipped before either eye but make no attempt to restore bifixation by convergence. Also, many orthophoric monofixating patients who have good acuity in each eye rapidly alternate their fixation to the uncovered eye as the prism is slipped before the fixating eye; consequently, neither eye shows a movement response.

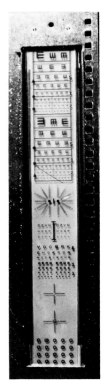

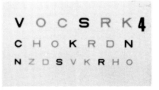
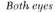

Both eyes

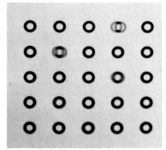

Range of stereoacuity (top to bottom): 240, 180, 120, 60, and 30 seconds of arc

VECTOGRAPHIC TEST FOR SUPPRESSION

Bifixation and monofixation are subtly determined in patients whose eyes appear straight by the A-O Vectographic Project-O-Chart Slide* used in conjunction with a nondepolarizing aluminized screen.* Each character on the slide has self-contained light polarizations, some polarized at 90° to others. Viewed through polaroid analysers, some images are visible to one eye and invisible to the other and some characters are visible to both eyes (Fig 9-12). This method provides a test environment closely approximating the normal binocular situation. The patient with bifixation reads the entire line of six 0.5 Snellen letters without hesitation, although two letters are seen only by the right eye, two others only by the left eye, and the remaining two letters by both eyes. The patient with monofixation deletes the two letters that are imaged only on the retina of the nonfixating eye. Occasionally, a patient with monofixation who rapidly alternates fixation from one eye to the other reads all six letters, but usually he comments that as two letters disappear, two others appear.

VECTOGRAPHIC TESTS FOR STEREOPSIS

Stereopsis is graded according to the least horizontal disparity in retinal image that evokes perception.

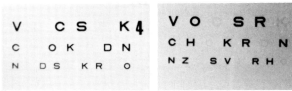

Right eye   *Left eye*

Fig 9-12. Polaroid vectographic slide (American Optical Company).

* American Optical Company.

The determination of stereoacuity is measured in seconds of arc of image disparity. Polaroid vectographs produce the image disparity, and the patient sees them through Polaroid analysers in normal room illumination. If the patient wears glasses, the analysers are fitted over them. The stereoacuity is measurable at either 6 meters or 40 cm.

Near stereoacuity is measured by either the Titmus Stereotest† (Fig 8-5) or the Wirt Stereotest‡ (Fig 5-14). The fly of the Titmus Stereotest produces approximately 3,000 seconds of arc of retinal image disparity at 40 cm. The Wirt Stereotest presents a range of stereotargets producing retinal image disparity between 1,000 and 14 seconds of arc at 40 cm, compared with the range of 800 to 40 seconds of arc at 40 cm for the Titmus Stereotest.

Distant stereoacuity is measured by the A-O Vectographic Project-O-Chart Slide (Fig 9-12) that presents a range of stereotargets between 30 and 240 seconds of arc at 6 meters.

---

† Stereotest, Titmus Optical Company.

‡ No longer available commercially.

Patients with central fusion have 40 seconds of arc or better at near (average of 24 seconds of arc on the Wirt Stereotest) and 30 seconds of arc at distance. Patients with peripheral fusion who lack central fusion have poorer stereoacuity scores, ranging from 3,000 to 60 seconds of arc at near (averaging 200 seconds of arc) and from 240 to 120 seconds of arc at distance. Stereoacuity is a very reliable and rapid method for screening patients to determine bifixation and monofixation. Patients having greater than 8Δ of horizontal deviation by simultaneous prism and cover and having ARC-type single binocular vision (demonstrated either by Worth 4 dots or by Bagolini striated lenses) do not appreciate stereopsis on the Stereo Fly Test, even when it is held only 20 cm from the eyes (approximately 6,000 seconds of arc). This supports the contention that ARC fusion is devoid of stereopsis. Stereopsis appears to be a binocular visual function that exists only in NRC if one accepts the thesis that peripheral NRC fusion can exist in patients having as much as 8Δ of horizontal deviation as disclosed by simultaneous prism and cover tests. According to this thesis, recognition of stereopsis is evidence that NRC fusion prevails, and the stereoacuity differentiates bifixation from monofixation.

10

Amblyopia

The fixation reflex must be developed and used until a child reaches approximately 9 years of age; otherwise, amblyopia will occur. Amblyopia in infants and children occurs commonly in strabismus unless the fixation is alternated from eye to eye. The unused eye of the young, nonalternating strabismic patient is deprived of fortifying the neurophysiologic activity involved in fixation; as a result, the cortical function of foveal discrimination is impaired. The degree of impairment of fixation is determined by the interplay of many factors. However, amblyopia is a deprivation phenomenon caused by not using the fixation reflex. It is related neither to the sensorial adaptations occurring in acquired strabismus nor to the absence of binocular vision found in congenital strabismus. It is a monocular problem and unrelated to the status of the binocular vision.

Burian (1) states that the clinician views amblyopia as being governed by two concepts: suppression and nonuse.

SUPPRESSION

Suppression is an active cortical inhibition of retinal innervations reaching the brain that subserves photopic form vision. This function is essentially macular; consequently, the implied cortical suppression affects innervational dispatches from primarily the macular and paramacular retinal areas. The cortical suppression must be very selective because it (1) develops only in young children, (2) functions during monocular seeing, (3) allows light discrimination to function normally, (4) affects form vision, (5) is confined to the photopic visual state, and (6) is confined to the macular and paramacular areas.

Suppression is one of the two adaptations in binocular vision that are discussed in the chapter titled Sensorial Adaptations in Strabismus. The term suppression, as it was used there, describes an active cortical inhibition of the visual impression arriving at the brain from the region of the retina of the deviated eye that receives the images from the area of conscious regard. Suppression also is a cortical process affecting a restricted region of the retina of one eye; however, unlike the suppression concept used to explain amblyopia, suppression to eliminate diplopia exists only during binocular viewing. For convenience, one will be referred to as "binocular suppression" and the other as "monocular suppression." Since monocular and binocular suppression are separate entities, one would expect the pathophysiology of each to be unrelated. Both forms develop only in the young, immature cortex. Either monocular or binocular suppression may exist alone, or they may coexist. Both may be either partially or totally overcome by treatment, but the treatment of one does not necessarily affect the other. The monocular suppression of amblyopia does not reduce the macular function to zero; although form perception of the macula may be impaired, the macular perception of light and color remains unimpaired. An absolute macular scotoma is not produced by monocular suppression. This contrasts to the absolute scotoma plottable during binocular perimetry that is produced by binocular suppression.

NONUSE

The most plausible explanation for amblyopia is that impairment of form vision results from lack of continuous attention to the images on each fovea. Exclusive attention to one foveal-cortical system and disuse of the other either prevents equal development of the normal fixation reflex of both eyes or allows one of the two normal fixation reflex systems to become less efficient than the other. The nonuse concept, better expressed by the term amblyopia exanopsia, has much to recommend it. Even if the active inhibitional process involved in suppressing form vision stimuli is accepted as the explanation for amblyopia, the essential condition that initiates such a neuropathophysiologic process is nonuse of the foveal-cortical system of one eye. The disuse concept implies that for the macular area to become permanently established as the retinal region which provides superior photopic form vision, it must be used for this purpose from infancy through 9 years of age. Discontinuing use of the fixation reflex after 9 years of age does not result in a lessening of its efficiency, but interruption of the use of this reflex at a younger age does reduce the quality of the reflex. Therefore, the nonuse concept suggests the following: (1) the foveal-cortical system is labile during the first nine years of life, requiring continuous conditioning before becoming a fixed, stable system; (2) monocular suppression of a normal foveal-cortical system is not required to produce amblyopia; and (3) consequently, amblyopia is simply the result of the child not using the foveal-cortical system adequately during its labile period.

Clinical and laboratory evidence supports nonuse as an explanation for amblyopia. Simply covering the eye of a child produces amblyopia in a very few weeks; in infants this occurs within days. Why would the cortex erect a complicated active inhibition system when no troublesome symptoms are produced by the child's occluded eye? The development of binocular suppression is an understandable response to the annoyance of diplopia after the onset of strabismus in a child with single binocular vision. It is rewarding to the patient to have the cortex eliminate the diplopia, but how does amblyopia reward the patient?

Covering the child's eye (or sealing the eyes of a newborn kitten, as performed by Hubel and Wiesel [2] to produce amblyopia is not equivalent to strabismus producing amblyopia because in the latter, light and image patterns continue to project into the deviated eye. Yet, it is for this reason that the suppression concept to explain amblyopia in strabismus has appeal. It could be argued that in strabismus, visual confusion results from dissimilar images projecting onto the two foveas. However, as described in the chapter Single Binocular Vision, a physiologic foveal scotoma appears in the deviated eye as soon as the strabismus begins, since the simultaneous perception of dissimilar images projecting onto the fovea is physiologically impossible. With a physiologic mechanism that prevents foveal visual confusion, it is difficult to accept the need for an elaborate cortical suppression system to develop a pathologic macular scotoma to eliminate the confusion. However, conceding the fact that the macular suppression of photopic form vision is demonstrable in the amblyopic eye, at most it would be a pathologic relative scotoma, and could not simple nonuse of the foveal-cortical system cause this finding?

ECCENTRIC FIXATION

Neither the suppression nor the nonuse concept explains the relative localization difficulties encountered in some patients whose amblyopia is severe enough to cause eccentric fixation. When the fixation capability of the fovea is so impaired that when the patient is forced to rely on this eye, better form vision is obtained by using the retina eccentric to the fovea, eccentric fixation is present. Normally the fovea is the zero straight-ahead reference point; however, this is altered in eccentric fixation, and the extramacular area of the retina chosen to receive the object of regard becomes the zero reference point. Rather than reason that a change occurred in the psycho-optic system controlling this relative localization function, von Noorden (3) credits Bielschowsky and Cuppers with adopting the view that eccentric fixation develops on the basis of anomalous retinal correspondence (ARC) and that this is the source of the altered relative localization. They believe the rearrangement of the visual directions in ARC during binocular viewing are carried over into monocular viewing. Von Noorden refuted this concept with visuscopic analysis of the eccentric fixation pattern, finding little correlation between the ARC angle of anomaly and the retinal region habitually chosen for eccentric fixation.

Although many questions about eccentric fixation remain unanswered, evidence is largely against its being related to ARC. However, one outstanding fact recurs often enough to make it difficult to totally dismiss the correspondence theory: during the treatment of eccentric fixation by pleoptics, monocular diplopia within the treated eye or binocular triplopia may transiently appear.

ACUITY

The difference in the acuity of the amblyopic eye for isolated letters and for whole-line letters is widely recognized. The fact that the acuity drops according to the degree the letters are crowded together is the crowding phenomenon. There is no satisfactory explanation for this phenomenon, but possibly it is a retinal, rather than a cortical, occurrence. As the amblyopia responds to treatment, the crowding phenomenon also reduces or vanishes. It is a more sensitive indicator of amblyopia than the acuity obtained on isolated letters; consequently, it has real therapeutic importance.

The visual acuity of the amblyopic eye corresponds roughly to the acuity of the normal eye at scotopic and mesopic luminance levels but is reduced at the photopic level. In fact, Burian (1) postulates that the cone system of the amblyopic eye acts as though the scotopic state is maintained during photopic luminance. Oculographic recordings have demonstrated an increase in the unsteadiness of fixation of the amblyopic eye in the photoptic state and a return to normal steadiness of fixation in the scotopic state. The electroretinogram and electroencephalogram have not been refined sufficiently to be acceptable tools in investigation of amblyopia.

DIAGNOSTIC TECHNIQUES

The definitive method for testing form acuity is to evaluate the patient's ability to discern increasingly small symbols. However, there are many instances in which a technique that grades the fixation reflex is substituted, allowing the examiner to draw inferences as to whether the form acuity is satisfactory from the patient's response; this is an indirect method of measuring the acuity.

DIRECT TESTING

Essentially the technique for directly testing vision entails showing a series of various-sized symbols at a fixed distance from the patient's eye and determining the smallest size that the patient can identify.

Snellen Test Type

The Snellen letters and illiterate E's are standard for measuring visual acuity. They are graded according to the angle they project at the nodal point of the eye. They are available for both distance and near testing and include symbols for testing both literates and illiterates. Intelligent and well-adjusted children of approximately 4 years of age are usually willing to try to perform at a level that permits a subjective evaluation of the acuity. Occasionally there is an exceptional child in whom acuity can successfully be determined between 3 and 4 years of age. If the patient is at the level that permits subjective evaluation of the acuity but is not literate, the examiner should use the Snellen illiterate E symbols for illiterates.

The ability to discern a group of symbols as contrasted to an isolated symbol varies according to the degree of amblyopia. In fact, a minimally amblyopic eye may identify isolated symbols almost as well as the nonamblyopic eye, but a significant difference of vision between the two is evident on viewing groups of symbols. Therefore, a line of symbols should always be offered to the patient, rather than just one symbol.

Another consistent difference between the eye with minor amblyopia and the normal eye is the ability to count symbols. Although the symbols are unidentifiable due to their small size, the normal eye rapidly and accurately counts lines of them; however, the amblyopic eye slowly and inaccurately counts lines of symbols that are large enough to be identified. For example, the best acuity of the good eye is 1.0, but the seven small symbols of the 1.5 line are accurately counted quickly and with little effort. The best acuity of the amblyopic eye is 0.6, and even with considerable effort and great pause, this eye is likely to obtain an incorrect count of the symbols in the 0.6, the 0.5, or even the 0.4 line.

Another distinction between normal and amblyopic eyes was shown by von Noorden and Burian (4). They demonstrated that when the intensity of illumination entering an eye is diminished by a neutral density filter placed before it, the acuity of the eye drops, according to the density of the filter. The same density filter that lowers the acuity in the normal eye by three or four lines has little or no effect on the visual acuity of the amblyopic eye. It is as though the amblyopic eye is in a state of relative dark adaptation compared with the fellow eye, and reduction of the illumination entering it does not influence its form perception. For example, if the best acuity is 1.0 in the right eye and 0.4 in the left eye, the best acuity in each is 0.4 through a neutral density filter of a certain value. Since the acuity of the poorer eye does not drop proportionately with the acuity of the better eye, the amblyopia is functional (amblyopia ex anopsia) rather than organic.

Landolt Ring

Symbols other than the Snellen letters and Snellen illiterate E's are available; the Landolt ring is of particular interest. This target is a ring with a sector missing, resembling the letter C (Fig 10-1). The break in the ring is oriented in various directions, and the patient identifies the target by specifying which part of the ring is missing. The beauty of this target is its uniformity as contrasted to the alphabet; this attribute is shared with the Snellen illiterate E.

Pictures

Pictures are another symbol available for illiterates (Fig 10-1). They are intended to project angles at the nodal point, equivalent to the Snellen symbols of comparable size; however, their varied shapes do not permit the same accuracy. The picture method should be reserved for those patients unable to be tested with the Snellen illiterate E method. How-

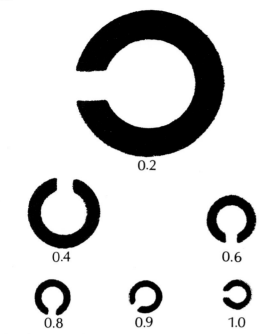

Fig 10-1. Landolt rings.

ever, usually the child who performs well on the pictures also does well with the Snellen illiterate E's. The picture material is a problem for some young children either because they have no personal experience with the article pictured or because they are unable to recall the noun. These factors are nonexistent in the Snellen illiterate E test.

INDIRECT TESTING

By testing the fixation reflex some conclusions may be made regarding visual acuity. The fixation reflex is investigated by a technique which evaluates the ability to align the eye so that the object of regard is projected on the retinal area having the maximal resolving power.

Cover-Uncover Test

The basic method of testing the fixation reflex is some variation of the cover-uncover test (Fig 6-1). Beginning with both eyes uncovered, the examiner places an occluder over one eye while he watches the uncovered eye. The critical time to closely observe the uncovered eye is the moment at which the cover is placed over the opposite eye. The examiner must be alert to any movement by the uncovered eye to fixate the object of regard. The cover is then removed, and the eyes are permitted to assume their original position; after a few moments, the

cover is placed over the other eye. If neither eye shifts when the cover is placed before the opposite eye, then either each is fixating foveally or the fixation is eccentric and steady in the one amblyopic eye.

This test is performed in lieu of a better method for evaluating the vision of infants, young children, and the mentally retarded, ie, those in whom testing by the Snellen test for illiterates is not feasible. An absence of movement of either eye during the cover-uncover test poses the problem as to whether the lack of movement is due to foveal fixation by each eye or to foveal fixation in one eye and eccentric fixation in the other; fortunately, there are two features that aid in differentiation between the two. Because strabismus is a prevalent cause of amblyopia in this age-group and if the deviation is large enough to be apparent, the eye with eccentric fixation may be revealed by persistence of its deviation when the preferred eye is covered. Another factor that aids in the differentiation of foveal and eccentric fixation is the reaction of the patient when the good eye is covered. If interest in the target material is maintained, the almost inevitable response is an attempt to evade an occluder before the good eye; there is no such evasive tactic when the bad eye is covered. Therefore, if a conspicuous deviation does not persist or if no objection is apparent on covering either eye, then the examiner may conclude, for want of better proof, that an absence of movement of either eye signifies an intact fixation reflex in both eyes. Consequently, the vision is judged to be satisfactory in each eye.

If one eye moves when the other is covered, the examiner must evaluate the ability of this eye to continue fixation after the removal of the cover. For example, if the right eye is the preferred eye and if when it is covered the strabismic left eye moves to take up fixation, the examiner must then determine what happens when the cover is removed from the right eye, ie, if the left eye continues fixation or if the right eye immediately reassumes fixation when the cover is lowered. If the left eye continues fixation, the deduction is that there is no difference between the acuity of the right and left eyes. However, if fixation of the left eye is invariably surrendered on removal of the cover over the right eye, then there is the possibility that, at the very least, the left eye is amblyopic relative to the right eye. True, this test does not quantitate the amblyopia of the left eye, but it does identify the poorer eye. If either strabismic eye continues steady fixation on the object of regard following removal of the cover, the inference is that the acuity is equal for each.

Since the cover-uncover test is used for infants, small children, and the mentally deficient, some consideration should be given to the nature of the occluder used by the examiner as well as to the fixation object selected for the test. Many of these patients are inordinately apprehensive and refuse to permit an occluder to approach their face. A more subtle covering technique may be necessary, and the examiner's thumb is probably the best substitute (Fig 10-2). Once the left hand is positioned lightly on the patient's head, the thumb is casually lowered in front of one eye and the cover-uncover test carried out. The examiner's right hand is occupied with pointing at the distant object of regard or holding a near fixation target. A running commentary about some feature of the fixation target is another essential component of the act. A light may be a successful fixation target at near but seldom is of any value at distance. A better distance target is a projected vision chart kept moving by either the examiner or a parent turning the knob on the projector which simulates television. A colorful, moving, music-playing toy at a distance is even better. Small pictures on tongue depressors and small toys attract attention at near for the brief period necessary to evaluate the fixation reflex. Infants and children should be seated on the parent's lap for this examination.

Visuscope

A more refined objective technique for studying the fixation reflex is to observe the retinal position of the projected target viewed by the patient within an ophthalmoscope beam. The instrument manufactured for this purpose is called the visuscope; a satisfactory homemade visuscope may be made from almost any ophthalmoscope.

The visuscope beam is directed through the dilated pupil, and the patient fixates the target outlined by the illumination system of the instrument (Fig 10-3). It is preferable to keep the illumination intensity reduced and also to use the red-free filter. The ophthalmoscopist judges to the accuracy of the foveal fixation, the ease with which it is established, and the rapidity with which it follows movement of the target. Gross inability to fixate foveally is easily ascertained. The eccentric fixation may obviously be at some point far from the fovea, and during this abortive fixation attempt the eye either constantly roams about a circumscribed area or is relatively still. As long as the eccentricity of fixation is paramacular or worse, judgments can be made with confidence. However, fixation errors of such small magnitude that the target moves about the macular area produce uncertainty in the mind of the examiner. There is a question as to whether the patient is seriously making the effort to foveally fixate or if he is incapable of accurate fixation; in great part, this question is answered by comparing the fixation pattern with that of the opposite eye. Another difficulty with this technique is the fact that some patients with proven excellent acuity and steady visuscopic fixation persistently keep the target slightly displaced from the center of the fovea. These factors make it difficult to judge any given eye, without knowing the visual acuity, as having absolute sustained foveal fixation ability or as having some deficiency in the fixation which is slightly less than foveal. Therefore, this technique admirably confirms grossly eccentric fixation but lacks the sensitivity to absolutely confirm perfect foveal fixation.

Visuscopy demands that the patient comprehend the directions to fixate and follow the target plus that he have the motivation to seriously cooperate. This is not a test of vision applicable to infants, young children, and the mentally defective. Generally, until the patient will cooperate in allowing his vision to be measured by the Snellen method for illiterates, he is an unlikely candidate for visuscopy.

Fig 10-2. Thumb occluder.

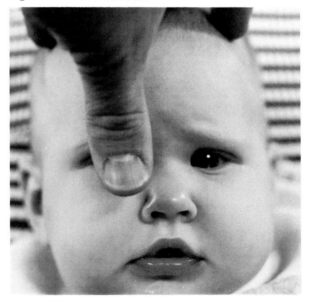

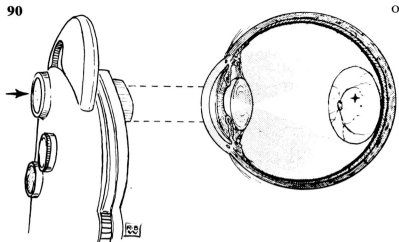

Fig 10-3. Visuscope.

Haidinger's Brushes

Since the entoptic phenomenon of Haidinger's brushes is appreciated only by a macular area with its center located at the fovea, an excellent system is available to check foveal fixation. Viewing polarized blue light through a rotating Nicol prism, the patient with macular function sees black, spinning Haidinger's brushes, resembling a whirling airplane propeller. The explanation of this entoptic phenomenon is probably related to the doubly refracting lutein of the macula, although it was previously thought to be caused by the polarizing action of the parallel arrangement of the Henle radial fibers at the fovea. The brushes are presented separately to each eye at approximately 40 cm, using the Coordinator* (Fig 10-4), and the patient is queried concerning his recognition of a spinning airplane propeller. The brushes vary in size according to the viewing distance from the source: the less the distance, the larger are the brushes, and vice versa. The patient may be asked to touch the center (better expressed by the word "hub") of the spinning propeller with a stylet. This presents no problem if the foveal fixation reflex is normal; if it is lacking, a gross error is surprisingly evident to the patient by the fact that the stylet point consistently misses the hub. This is due to the fact that the retinal projection of the stylet point is located on an extrafoveal point while the hub of the Haidinger's brushes is located on the fovea. The hub of the propeller is seen at the point at which the fixation axis intersects the viewing surface, which is displaced away from the extrafoveally fixated stylet point. Nasal eccentric fixation, typically found in esotropia, is associated with a nasal mislocation of the propeller

* Oculus.

hub in relation to the stylet point, whereas temporal eccentric fixation, more commonly encountered in exotropia, causes an erroneous positioning of the propeller temporally. Vertical discrepancies between propeller hub and stylet point mixed with the horizontal are not unusual.

Once the error between stylet point and propeller hub is recognized, the immediate reflex is to correct the error; consequently, a quick adjustment is made in the stylet position. However, the result of this move causes frustration and disbelief: no matter how the stylet is moved, the hub of the propeller moves accordingly. This is due to the fact that the eccentric retinal point continues to view the stylet point no matter where it is moved and therefore the fixation axis moves accordingly, with a proportionate change in the location of the brushes.

To use a technique encompassing eye and hand coordination, a transparent slide with an airplane drawn on it can be placed over the polarized illuminated plate of the Coordinator. The patient touches the stylet point on a center spot of the airplane engine which coincides with the point where the propeller hub should be located. Using the hand strengthens fixation and discourages the patient from reflexly making a corrective repositioning of the eccentrically fixating eye. This assists the examiner in questioning the patient in detail about the location of the brushes in regard to the eccentric fixation point (Fig 10-4).

Patients with large degrees of fixation eccentricity are unable to appreciate the brushes because the fixation axis misses the illuminated test plate of the instrument. Bringing the patient's face closer to the plate and thus reducing the viewing distance may prevent the angle of eccentricity from interfering with the patient seeing the brushes; this tech-

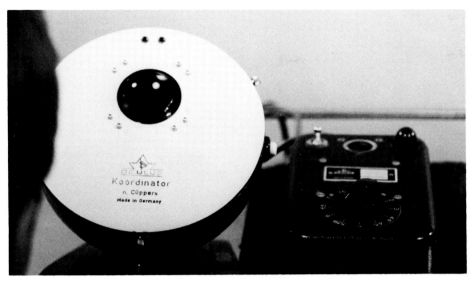

Fig 10-4. Coordinator (Oculus).

nique solves the problem for some, but not all. The patient should fixate the instrument with his good eye first in order to know what he is searching for with the amblyopic eye.

The Haidinger's brushes test for foveal fixation requires a good deal of maturity. A child must be a keen observer with a good attention span and must be able to clearly verbalize his experiences. The test is seldom useful in patients under 7 years of age.

REFERENCES

1. Burian HM: Pathophysiologic basis of amblyopia and its treatment. Am J Ophthalmol 67:1, 1969

2. Hubel DH, Wiesel TH: Single-cell response in striate cortex of kittens deprived of vision in one eye. J Neurophysiol 26:1003, 1963

3. von Noorden GK: The etiology and pathogenesis of fixation anomalies in strabismus. Trans Am Ophthalmol Soc 67:698, 1969

4. von Noorden GK, Burian HM: Visual acuity in normal and amblyopic patients under reduced illumination: I. Behavior of visual acuity with and without neutral density filter. Arch Ophthalmol 61:533, 1959

11

Treatment of the Sensorial Adaptations and Amblyopia

Suppression, anomalous retinal correspondence (ARC), and amblyopia are preventable in most strabismus patients by instituting the appropriate therapy at the correct time and closely following the patient during the first 10 years of life. Prophylaxis of the sensorial adaptations and amblyopia is ideal; however, the ophthalmologist does not always have the opportunity to apply the ideal, or he may not always find it practical. Patients with congenital constant strabismus persisting with growth do not develop suppression and ARC since they are devoid of single binocular vision; only patients who develop single binocular vision prior to the onset of their strabismus develop suppression and ARC. Thus, prophylaxis of these sensorial adaptations is directed only to patients who acquire strabismus during the first decade of life. Even if the strabismus is intermittent, these adaptations may develop in the patient with acquired strabismus; therefore, it is less than ideal to defer prophylactic therapy until the strabismus becomes constant.

Unlike suppression and ARC, amblyopia may develop in both patients with congenital strabismus and patients with acquired strabismus. Statistically, it is less likely to occur in patients whose strabismus is congenital than in those with acquired strabismus; among the patients with acquired strabismus it is rare in intermittent tropia but common in constant tropia.

The prophylactic therapy of suppression, ARC, and amblyopia may be either passive or active.

Passive prophylactic therapy entails occluding first one eye and then the other on alternate days. Alternate occlusion eliminates diplopia and visual confusion and ensures equal fixation time with each macula. In patients with congenital strabismus it is beneficial only if the patient does not spontaneously alternate the fixation from eye to eye; if indicated, it should be started by 6 months of age. In patients with acquired intermittent strabismus it is contraindicated because occlusion reduces the tone in the fusional vergence system that is so necessary to compensate for the deviation. Therefore, although occlusion as passive prophylactic therapy in intermittent strabismus may prevent suppression, ARC, and amblyopia on the one hand, on the other hand it increases the risk of the intermittent tropia deteriorating to a constant tropia. Thus, occlusion therapy in intermittent strabismus may be more harmful than helpful. Furthermore, most patients with intermittent strabismus bifixate sufficiently to prevent the development of amblyopia, so alternate occlusion to prevent amblyopia is rarely required. Patients with acquired constant strabismus always benefit from the alternate occlusion therapy if a more positive therapeutic approach is impossible. Ideally, the occlusion is applied during the entire period the patient is awake.

Active prophylactic therapy is either something that straightens the strabismic eyes or something that prismatically compensates for the strabismic angle. Surgery, lenses, or miotics may straighten the eyes; whatever the treatment, it must be applied shortly after the onset of the strabismus and must be sufficient to totally straighten the eyes to qualify as prophylactic therapy. Partially reducing the strabismic angle and leaving a residual deviation falls short of offering active prophylaxis against the development of suppression, ARC, and amblyopia.

It is evident that the ideal treatment of strabismus in children carries with it a degree of urgency. Delaying the institution of the prophylactic therapy is less than ideal strabismus management.

SUPPRESSION

It is feasible to induce the cortex to terminate the use of the active inhibitory reflex it developed to free the strabismic patient of diplopia. Some patients succeed in overcoming the suppression, but others fail. The patient must have concentration and motivation in order to succeed. However, apart from this, there is a fundamental difference in the ease with which esotropic patients overcome suppression as compared with exotropic patients. Many exotropes apparently have a more profound suppression than esotropes, and no matter what degree of effort is applied, exotropes often never achieve diplopia recognition. Perhaps this is due to the difference in the suppression between the nasal and the temporal retina.

One method of overcoming suppression is to place a red filter before one eye, producing dissimilarly colored images when the patient fixates a light. He is instructed to fixate either the red or the white image but at the same time try to see the other image. When the deviated eye is rapidly covered and uncovered with an occluder, the previously suppressed image now may be seen alternately with the first. For patients unable to recognize diplopia by this method, a 15Δ prism is placed vertically before the deviating eye. In esotropes this usually displaces the image out of the suppression scotoma, and diplopia is immediately apparent. Exotropes may not be so quick to recognize diplopia; in this case, it helps to wiggle the prism, constantly moving the image that is flashing on and off on the suppressed temporal retina as the therapist rapidly covers and uncovers the eye. As diplopia is gradually recognized, the patient should concentrate on maintaining it. Next, the red filter is removed, and it is hoped that the patient now continues to see two different white lights alternately flashing on and off. The movement of the occluder is stopped, and again two sustained lights should be maintained. If the vertical prism was necessary, it is withdrawn either abruptly or gradually; now the two lights are maintained, and the patient is taught to transfer fixation of the light from eye to eye, maintaining diplopia while either eye fixates. After accomplishing diplopia, the patient should recognize first a light and then contoured targets (eg, a doorknob or a light switch) as diplopic. As soon as the patient's attention wanes, suppression returns. With great concentration he may momentarily recall diplopia. Occlusion is continued when diplopia recognition is not being exercised, to prevent renewal of the habit of suppression.

The orthoptist may use the major amblyoscope rather than the fixation light, red filter, occluder, and vertical prism to conduct the antisuppression treatment. The tubes are set at zero, and as the patient alternates his fixation on the target, he gradually becomes momentarily aware of the blurred peripheral image in the nonfixating eye. The examiner encourages this awareness by flashing and oscillating the tube containing the target projected into the nonfixating eye. When the patient recognizes diplopia on the machine, then he practices on regular targets in everyday seeing as previously described.

ANOMALOUS RETINAL CORRESPONDENCE

Once the patient recognizes diplopia and ARC is apparent, then the orthoptist attempts to awaken normal retinal correspondence (NRC) by either prismatically compensating for the angle or placing the amblyoscope tubes at the objective setting. As the patient concentrates on fusing the identical targets or on superimposing the large, dissimilar targets, the single image in the nonfixating eye intermittently may be momentarily recognized as double. This is monocular diplopia or binocular triplopia and represents a transient stage the patient experiences as ARC and NRC vie with one another to localize the image in the nonfixating eye. Once the patient fuses with NRC, occlusion of one eye is maintained while he is not undergoing orthoptic therapy so the habits of suppression and using ARC are prevented. This is maintained until the alignment of the eyes is straightened by surgery or is compensated for by prisms.

In North America, orthoptic therapy for suppression and ARC has nearly vanished. The decline has resulted from a change in the previous viewpoint that orthoptic therapy prior to surgery increased the percentage of good results from that of surgery alone. Strabismic patients with suppression and ARC spontaneously adjust these sensorial adaptations postsurgically to conform to the new alignment. If straight eyes are surgically achieved, the patient returns to NRC. However, if constant strabismus was preoperatively present for a month or more, the patient usually does not return to bifixation; instead, a macular scotoma is manifest in the nonfixating eye. Orthoptic therapy before and/or after surgery does not alter this outcome. No greater percentage of patients with constant strabismus bifixate after surgery by receiving therapy for suppression and ARC.

The best result a constantly strabismic patient with suppression and ARC can hope for is NRC peripheral fusion. Normal retinal correspondence is better than ARC because fusional vergence functions in NRC; this is necessary to keep the patient's eyes straight throughout his lifetime. There is no significant fusional vergence amplitude in ARC; whatever eye alignment change occurs through the years, the ARC and suppression also change accordingly, to conform to the angle of deviation. Thus, ARC has little or no influence on maintaining a constant alignment of the eyes throughout life. Since ARC therapy has not been shown to produce a better postoperative chance for NRC peripheral fusion with straight eyes, it is difficult to justify ARC therapy.

Patients with intermittent exotropia tend to develop profound suppression and ARC which prevail during the tropia phase only to be replaced by NRC central fusion as soon as the eyes come straight. Once the suppression and ARC have developed, the patient can always recall those cortical adaptations into use even though orthoptic therapy has taught him to avoid them. To prevent the natural and almost automatic assertion of suppression and ARC when the exodeviation occurs requires alertness, motivation to keep the eyes straight, and willingness to put forth the necessary effort. Orthoptic therapy is relatively successful in these patients, but eventually most patients tire of this ordeal and allow the intermittent exodeviation to return with its associated suppression and ARC. Orthoptic therapy for the sensorial adaptations in intermittent strabismus has not been proven to enhance the final postoperative result as compared with surgery without prior therapy.

AMBLYOPIA

Treatment of amblyopia is to force the patient to visually depend on the eye which has diminished acuity. The usual method of accomplishing this is to occlude the eye which has better acuity. However, there are alternate methods of limited value, ie, atropinization of the better eye and producing a state of relative hypofunction of the perimacular area of the amblyopic eye by dazzling it with a bright light.

OCCLUSION

Amblyopia therapy is indicated between 6 months and 9 years of age if the fixation of one eye is less than that of the other or if acuity is less than 20/30 (6/9).* Therapy is also advised to prevent restoration of amblyopia in a patient who has equal fixation or good visual acuity after occlusion therapy

* Metric equivalent given in parentheses after Snellen notation.

if the patient continues to fixate with the preferred eye and does not alternate. Part-time occlusion is prescribed in the latter case; otherwise, occlusion is used during the entire waking day. Total 24-hour occlusion is never used, as it can produce unimprovable amblyopia in a normal eye. The occluded eye is always allowed a few minutes of use each day when the patient first awakes and before he goes to bed. Occlusion for the entire waking day is very safe and effective therapy.

When occlusion is prescribed, it is always demonstrated to the parents on the patient. The parents are made to understand that the occlusion therapy is their responsibility. If the child pulls off the patch, they should deal with this forthright. Infants or very young children who pull at the occluding patch can be dissuaded from this by mittens; elbow restraints are used if everything else fails. The parent is told how to make the restraints using tongue depressors in flannel silverware wrappers. The restraints are tied above and below the elbow, allowing free use of the hands, wrists, and shoulders but preventing flexion of the elbow so the fingers cannot grasp the occluding patch. Usually the elbow restraints are required for no more than three days before the child accepts the occlusion.

In a patient 6 months of age, amblyopia can be overcome in three or four days, and the occluded eye becomes amblyopic; parents should be informed of this possibility and be made to understand that this is the therapeutic goal. The induced amblyopia can easily be overcome in a few days by reversing the occlusion. Because of the rapidity with which amblyopia is overcome in very young children, children under 1 year of age are reexamined within one week of starting occlusion; if they are between 1 and 2 years of age, they are reexamined in two weeks; and if they are over 2 years, they return routinely one month after starting occlusion. Since the fixation preference is switched in very young children from one eye to the other after a very few days of occlusion, prior to placing the occluder each morning, the mother should determine which eye is preferred by observing the reflected corneal image in reference to the pupillary center. An ignited match, cigarette lighter, or flashlight can be the source of the corneal reflection.

Patch

A patch that adheres to the skin around the eyelids is the method of occlusion for most children. Some older children favor a patch that is tied on or that is retained in position by an elastic tape encircling the skull; however removal is so easily accomplished by the patient that this method usually fails. Various adhesive occlusion materials are available that stick to the skin, thus discouraging removal by the patient. The two most widely used products in North America are the Elastoplast Eye Occlusors,* manufactured in junior and regular sizes, and the Opticlude Orthoptic Eye Patch,† manufactured in only one size. Occasionally a child is allergic to the adhesive in the Elastoplast, but the Opticlude is nonallergenic. Perspiration makes it difficult for the adhesive to adhere to the skin; the Opticlude is more successful than the Elastoplast in retaining adhesion. Tincture of benzoin applied to the skin prior to the eye patch helps solve the problem resulting from perspiration; it also forms a base on the skin that prevents the ulceration that occurs in some children. An excellent adhesive material is the Micropore† paper tape which is not loosened by perspiration and is nonallergenic; this can easily be fashioned into an occluder by cutting a 5-cm piece off the roll of tape (Fig 11-1).

Lens

Children usually accept lens occlusion (Fig 11-1) and do not pull the spectacles down to peek over the covered lens if the acuity in the amblyopic eye is better than 20/60 (6/18). This is the preferred occlusion technique for children who wear spectacles and who have an acuity of at least 20/50 (6/15). Spectacles are worn over the face occlusion if the amblyopia is more severe. The Lindner occluder‡ (Fig 11-2), which attaches to the back

Fig 11-1. Lens occlusion.

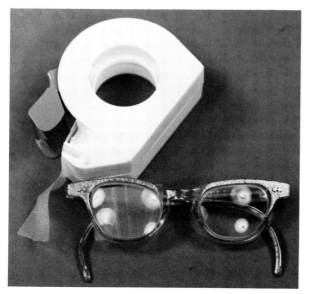

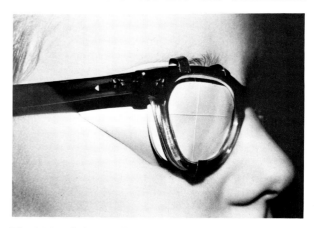

Fig 11-2. Lindner occluder (American Optical Company).

of the spectacle lens and is held in place against the face with the soft rubber rim sealing out light entering the occluded eye, is no better than simply covering the lens with tape.

Part-Time

Part-time occlusion usually consists of forced use of the nonpreferred eye for one half of each day. In school-age children it is conducted during the portion of the day spent outside school. Children who do not wear spectacles use the eye patch; those who do wear spectacles usually have the A-O occluder lens‡ (Fig 11-3) inserted in one pair of spectacles and have a second pair of spectacles with clear lenses. The great advantage of the A-O occluder lens is that the observer can see through it and is not aware that the eye is occluded. The patient can see no better than 20/800 (6/240) through the occluder lens, and since he has vision of 20/50 (6/15) or better in the nonpreferred eye, he readily chooses to fixate through the clear spectacle lens. The lens is available as either a plano power lens or a rough lens that allows a power to be ground on the front surface. Ideally, a power should be ground on the front surface to match the opposite lens in the spectacles if it has a power of 3 diopters or greater. With lens weights and with magnification or minification power being equal, the appearance of the spectacles is attractive. The frosted-lens or dimpled-lens occluders are unsightly

---

* Duke Laboratories, Stamford, Ct.

† Minnesota Mining.

‡ American Optical Company.

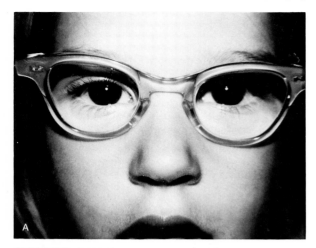

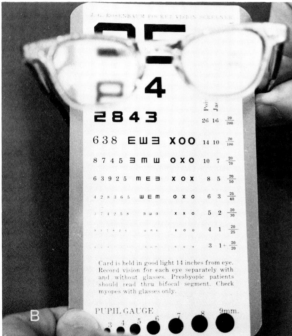

Fig 11-3. A. Occluder lens, left spectacle lens (American Optical Company). **B.** 20/800 (6/240) occluder lens, left spectacle lens.

compared with the excellent appearance of the A-O occluder lens. For children who need long-range part-time occlusion therapy, this technique has been eminently successful in maintaining high morale in both parents and children.

Contact Lenses

The author has used an occluder contact lens for many years in infants, most frequently in patients with aphakia or high-degree anisometropia. How-

ever, the hard contact lens is not a practical method for controlling strabismus amblyopia. Possibly the contact lens will become a practical occlusion method with development of a soft lens that covers the entire cornea and occludes the eye by virtue of its being opaque, providing it can be left in the eye safely throughout the entire waking day. The present hard occluder contact lens displaces easily; usually a portion of the pupillary space is visible around the periphery of the lens. A long-acting miotic instilled daily in the occluded eye helps to offset this complication. Despite this, some children rub the eye to dislodge the lens and gain use of the occluded eye. At any rate, this occlusion technique in its present form has not been universally successful.

Visuscopy reveals inaccuracies of foveal fixation, the retinal area the patient chooses for fixation when fixation is less than foveal, and grossly eccentric fixation in profound amblyopia. However, it has proven to be neither a better guide for assessing the results of occlusion therapy nor a better indicator for initiating occlusion therapy than the fixation test performed by cover-uncover or the determination of the visual acuity. Pleoptists claimed in the past that patients with eccentric fixation should have the eccentrically fixating eye occluded for a month or more to reduce the established pattern before initiation of occlusion of the preferred eye. The wisdom of this therapy has not been substantiated by clinical facts. Such a practice is of questionable value since it delays initiation of the positive therapy that overcomes amblyopia—occluding the preferred eye.

The objective of the occlusion therapy is to equalize the fixation skill or visual acuity in the two eyes. If the vision has not improved within six months, therapy is discontinued. When vision has maximally improved and occlusion therapy is terminated, there is approximately a 50-percent chance of restoration of amblyopia. Amblyopic patients almost never bifixate after their amblyopia is eradicated, despite glasses, surgery, prisms, miotics, orthoptics, or other treatment. If bifixation were obtainable, the amblyopia would not return. Since this result is not obtainable, then the only way to avoid the return of amblyopia is for the patient to adopt the habit of alternate fixation. This occurs in approximately half of the patients; however, just as frequently preference for one eye continues, causing amblyopia to return in the nonpreferred eye within one to three months. It is important to recognize the reappearance of amblyopia quickly and to initiate part-time occlusion. Once this trait is identified in a patient, the part-time occlusion is continued until he reaches 9 years of age. Thereafter, the visual acuity usually holds throughout life at the same level it was when occlusion therapy was discontinued.

ATROPINIZATION

Atropine instilled in the preferred eye is effective treatment only if the acuity in the amblyopic eye is 20/50 (6/15) or better; otherwise, the patient prefers the blurred image presented to the preferred eye. Also, the greater the degree of plus and cylinder refractive error in the preferred eye, the better it works. A 1% solution of atropine is instilled in the preferred eye each morning; if part-time occlusion is desired, it is instilled at weekly intervals. It is useful in the child who receives miotics for controlling esotropia, does not wear glasses, and has a recurrent amblyopia that is controlled by part-time occlusion. In this instance atropinization of the preferred eye and miotic therapy of the nonpreferred eye is a workable combination.

PLEOPTICS AND ORTHOPTICS

Another method to overcome amblyopia is a multiple approach with an array of aggressive techniques. It is designed to motivate the child to try harder to improve his fixation skill and to more rapidly improve the visual acuity in the nonpreferred eye. The final result in the majority of amblyopic patients is the same whether the less aggressive, simple occlusion therapy is used exclusively or if pleoptic exercises are used. An eccentrically fixating eye in some older children has been restored to central fixation using pleoptics after occlusion therapy has failed. This has usually required multiple and laborious exercises, which are built around a technique, designed by Bangerter in Switzerland, that dazzles the area of the retina surrounding the macula of the amblyopic eye with a strong light from an instrument called a pleoptophor. As soon as the intense light is turned off, the macula supposedly functions better than the surrounding hypofunctioning paramacular area. A similar technique known as euthyscopy, designed by Cüppers of Germany, dazzles the perimacular retinal area with intense light from a modified ophthalmoscope that incorporates an opaque disk in the light beam to protect the macula. As soon as the dazzling light is discontinued, the patient's attention is called to the afterimage; he is instructed to attempt to see using the macula, which is identified by its location in the center of the afterimage ring. The limited success of these techniques raises the practical question of whether it is worth the expense and trouble. For the eccentrically fixating patient who has lost use of the preferred eye, it certainly is worth it. Aside from this example, however, the question of the value of pleoptics remains. Ophthalmologists in North America have examined this issue and rejected pleoptics as a practical method of treating amblyopia.

Orthoptists have used hand-eye coordination exercises in the treatment of amblyopia for many years. For example, the amblyopic patient undergoing treatment wears a red filter before the preferred eye. The patient is to select red-and-white patterned material; this can be performed only with the nonpreferred eye since both the red and the white in the patterned material appear red to the eye behind the red filter. Stringing small red and white beads in sequence or tracing red and white patterns are basic orthoptic procedures for amblyopia. Orthoptists also have used the cheiroscope, which by its angled mirror septum allows only the preferred eye to fixate a picture that is traced by the amblyopic eye. Instruction in these exercises and checks on their progress are performed during office visits at designated intervals; however, the major work is done at home by the patient. Occlusion of the normal eye is continued while the patient is not doing the exercises.

The main contrast between the above-described orthoptic approach to amblyopia and the pleoptic approach from Switzerland and Germany is that European children are hospitalized and their treatment sessions are conducted twice daily by a trained staff. The pleoptic approach further includes the therapy with dazzling light. Between treatment sessions the amblyopic eye is usually occluded, rather than the preferred eye, to prevent the patient from reverting to the abnormal fixation habit. Once central fixation replaces eccentric fixation, the occlusion is transferred to the preferred eye.

12

Concomitant Esodeviations

Concomitant esodeviations are those in which the convergent angle of the eyes remains unchanged regardless of the direction of gaze; the alignment is the same in the primary position, lateral gaze, and vertical gaze. Concomitant esodeviations are caused by or associated with various unrelated factors such as the near reflex, a congenital hypertonus of the medial recti, an acquired hypotonus of the lateral recti and unilateral reduced visual function in an infant or young child.

ACCOMMODATIVE ESODEVIATIONS

A convergent deviation of the eyes associated with activation of the accommodation reflex is an accommodative esodeviation. If the accommodative esodeviation is within the fusional divergence amplitude, it is accommodative esophoria; however, if the accommodative esodeviation is beyond the scope of fusion, it is accommodative esotropia.

ETIOLOGY

Either of two separate causes, or a combination of the two, precipitates accommodative esotropia. The first cause is, as Donders described, the convergence associated with accommodation applied to clear the blurred retinal image caused by hypermetropia. If the retinal image is allowed to remain blurred, the hypermetropic patient is not accommodating and the eyes remain straight. However, clearing the blurred hypermetropic image is accomplished by accommodation, and there is also a synkinetic accommodative esodeviation.

The second cause of accommodative esodeviation is a high accommodative convergence to accommodation (AC/A) ratio (see chapter entitled Vergences). In patients with normal refractions, an abnormal relationship between accommodation and its synkinetically associated accommodative convergence can cause an esodeviation at near. The amount of convergence associated with each diopter of accommodation may vary from slight to marked. Also, a patient may have both hypermetropia and a high AC/A ratio.

In children, accommodative esophoria is usually asymptomatic. If a symptom appears, it is usually asthenopia which occurs after prolonged near work. As the fusional divergence fatigues, controlling the esophoria by maintaining fusion becomes increasingly difficult. Eventually, esotropia momentarily replaces esophoria, and the patient experiences diplopia. The diplopia causes the patient to react by reducing the accommodation, hence lessening the associated accommodative convergence which reduces the esophoria to the level at which the fatigued fusional divergence can regain fusion. Esotropia returns to esophoria, but the retinal image is blurred due to underaccommodation and, as a consequence, visual acuity is reduced. The reduced acuity stimulates the patient to increase the accommodation which, in turn, causes return of the diplopia. This recurrent cycle of diplopia vacillating with blurred vision is often experienced by the fatigued esophoric patient. Patients with accommodative esophoria caused by a high AC/A ratio have these symptoms at near, whereas those with accommodative esophoria caused by hypermetropia have symptoms at both distance and near.

The onset of accommodative esotropia may occur at any age between 6 months and 7 years; the average age of the patient at onset is 2½ years, regardless of the cause. Apparently, this is the usual age at which the youngster first accommodates sufficiently to appreciate the visual gain, although he experiences diplopia. He does not sustain the accommodation, but the recurring esotropia produces the clinical pattern of intermittent esotropia. Attention to fine visual detail causes momentary esotropia at both distance and near if hypermetropia is the cause and only at near if a high AC/A ratio is the cause. Some patients maintain the intermittent esotropia pattern without manifestations of an increase toward constant esotropia; however, others increase the frequency and duration of esotropia and rapidly convert to constant esotropia.

The causes of accommodative esotropia are hereditary, as manifest by the patient with siblings, a parent, or multiple other relatives with the same disorder.

CLINICAL INVESTIGATION

The clinical investigation of these patients demands an evaluation of the cycloplegic refraction, the AC/A ratio, and the fusional divergence amplitude because these three factors determine the cause of esodeviation and the patient's ability to contain the accommodative esodeviation and to maintain fusion.

An adequate cycloplegic refraction need not be atropine refraction. One drop of 2% cyclopentolate (Cyclogyl) within 40 minutes provides within 0.25 D of the plus refractive error produced by one drop of 1% atropine t.i.d. for three days in white children. Deeply pigmented irides require more than one drop of 2% cyclopentolate, ie, the addition of one drop of 10% phenylephrine hydrochloride (Neo-Synephrine), one drop of 1% atropine, and 40 minutes later one drop of 1% tropicamide (Mydriacyl). This produces superb cycloplegia one hour after the first drops are instilled in the most deeply pigmented eyes. Ideally, evaluation of the cycloplegic refraction should be included in the examination conducted during the initial appointment, and glasses if needed should be prescribed at the termination of this examination. Also, regardless of the cycloplegic drugs used in children, a certain residual hypermetropia remains. Repeat cycloplegic refraction within weeks after prescribing the first glasses usually discloses more hypermetropia than was detected at the initial refraction.

The AC/A ratio is determined by comparing the distance prism, near prism, and alternate cover accommodation controlled measurements (see chapter entitled Vergences). A near esodeviation measurement within 10Δ of the distance measurement is considered within the normal range. A high AC/A measurement has an excess of 10Δ difference between distance and near. Since the severity of the high AC/A measurement varies from patient to patient, the severity of the ratio is thus graded. Grade 1 high AC/A ratio includes the difference from 11Δ to 20Δ between the distance and near measurements; grade 2 is the difference from 21Δ through 30Δ; and grade 3 is the difference in excess of 30Δ. Infants and children fixate toys at distance and near as the prism and alternate cover measurements are performed. Children who submit to a visual acuity test with Snellen letters or the Snellen illiterate *E's* fixate the same targets for their distance–near testing. The lines of columns of letters are read as the cover test is performed on literate children, and illiterate children point out the direction of the E's which are continuously presented during cover testing.

TABLE 12-1. Relationship Between AC/A Ratio and Refraction in Patients With Accommodative Esotropia

Patients	AC/A	Refractions
378	Normal	+2.25
289	High	+4.75

Any combination of refraction and AC/A ratio can be found, but statistically there is a definite relationship. Patients with a normal AC/A ratio have relatively more hypermetropia, and those with a high AC/A ratio have relatively less hypermetropia. One study (1) reveals the relationships shown in Table 12-1. This is according to expectations since patients with a high AC/A ratio should have to accommodate less than patients with a normal AC/A ratio to produce equal angles of accommodative esodeviation.

The fusional divergence amplitude usually ranges between 12Δ and 20Δ; when the accommodative esodeviations exceed this range, esotropia prevails. By trial and error, the fusional divergence amplitude can be indirectly determined by doing the prism and alternate cover test while the patient is wearing the minimal hypermetropic lenses that permit fusion (see chapter entitled Vergences). Patients with accommodative esodeviation who remain intermittently esotropic for several years tend to maintain the largest fusional divergence amplitudes. The patient who lapses into constant esotropia soon loses the large fusional divergence amplitude previously possessed when the strabismus was intermittent.

Sensory and motor complications soon evolve if esotropia repeatedly vacillates with esophoria. Initially, diplopia is experienced when esotropia first appears; however, the young child soon learns suppression and adopts ARC (anomalous retinal correspondence) peripheral fusion, removing any sensory annoyances that occur during the esotropic phase. Until this happens, the child often manifests diplopia and visual confusion by expressing it verbally, by closing or covering one eye, and by his awkwardness. As soon as these sensory annoyances are eliminated by development of the sensorial adaptations, the patient is happier and more willing to tolerate the tropia. Eventually, constant esotropia may replace intermittent esotropia. After developing suppression and ARC and while still intermittently esotropic, when the eyes are straight, NRC (normal retinal correspondence) and central and peripheral fusion are present. Such patients instantly adjust their sensory status to conform to the alignment of the eyes.

A motor complication also occurs in intermittent esotropia; it is presumably a change in the medial recti secondary to their increased and more frequent contraction. Whatever this change, ie, hypertrophy or contracture, a gradual nonaccommodative esodeviation increase appears. Eventually, the non-accommodative esodeviation build-up exceeds the fusional divergence amplitude in most patients, and the intermittent esotropia is replaced by constant esotropia. As the angle of esotropia increases, the ARC values and localization of the suppression scotoma change accordingly to conform to the larger angle.

With constant esotropia comes an opportunity for amblyopia to develop. Most patients with acquired esotropia, in contrast to those with congenital esotropia, select their favorite eye for fixation to the exclusion of the other eye; this soon results in amblyopia of the unused eye. If, by chance, alternate fixation is chosen, amblyopia is prevented. Amblyopia is unrelated to suppression and ARC. While the intermittent phase of the accommodative esotropia prevails, suppression and ARC may begin; however, amblyopia may not begin because there is sufficient bifoveal fixation to prevent it. Only when constant esotropia replaces intermittent esotropia is the strabismus capable of causing the development of amblyopia in the patient with non-alternate fixation. However, suppression and ARC are always present in constant acquired esotropia, regardless of alternate or nonalternate fixation; they also occur during the intermittent esotropia phase.

TREATMENT

Early recognition of the disorder and early initiation of treatment are mandatory if the sensory and motor complications are to be prevented. The basic treatment involves some technique that curbs accommodation. This is accomplished by either an optic method (glasses) or instillation of a parasympathomimetic drug (miotic) into the eyes.

The treatment varies according to the patient's age when the ophthalmologist is first consulted. For convenience the treatment is described for three age-groups: children under 4 years, children between 4 and 8 years, and patients over 8 years.

Under 4 Years of Age

In all children under 4 years of age, the full cycloplegic refraction spectacle correction is prescribed (Fig 12-1). Occasionally, the history is not help-

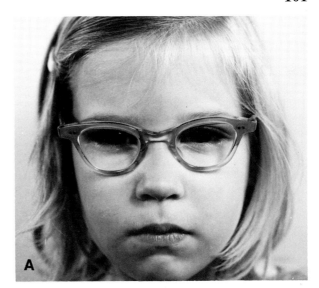

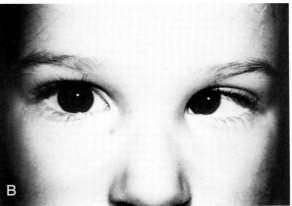

Fig 12-1. A. Straight eyes while large hypermetropic spectacle correction is worn. **B.** Accommodative esotropia when spectacles are removed.

ful, findings are rather questionable, and the ophthalmologist wishes to gain evidence regarding improvement in the angle of esotropia by curbing the accommodation, but he has reason to doubt whether or not glasses are important or perhaps the glasses are rejected despite all efforts to encourage acceptance, eg, instillation of 1% atropine each morning for one month. For whatever reason, it is helpful in these circumstances to prescribe instillation of a miotic each morning. The miotic should be considered as temporary therapy; it is to be used until the importance of the antiaccommodation element is determined or until the child has matured and accepts the needed glasses. Miotics should not be considered as alternative permanent antiaccommodation therapy equal to glasses.

The patient is reexamined at monthly intervals until the physician is certain that the glasses control the accommodative esotropia. If the esotropia remains at near but the eyes are straight at distance, an additional +2.50 D bifocal segment is prescribed (Fig 12-2). Care is taken to inform the optician that the top of the lower segment must be higher for children than for adults. Ideally, the top of the segment must be 3 mm above the 6-o'clock limbus position. Segments that are too low are either viewed over or the child must raise the chin too high in order to depress the eyes to see through the segments. If the optician places the top of the segment too high, the bifocals will be higher than midpupil, causing the chin to be depressed while viewing at distance through the upper portion of the bifocals. Children who do not readily accept the lower segment for near viewing and continue to cross their eyes for near viewing while look-

Fig 12-2. A. High AC/A ratio causing near esotropia despite fully corrective distance hypermetropic spectacles. **B.** Bifocal segment adds compensation for the high AC/A ratio, permitting straight eyes for near viewing.

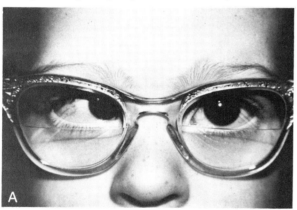

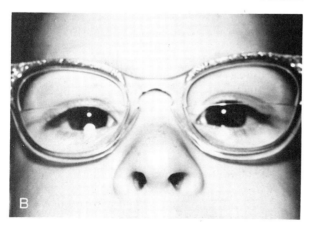

ing through the upper portions of the lenses are started on 1% atropine instillation daily. This therapy is continued for one month. After the atropine is discontinued, the child usually continues to use the lower segment correctly. The ophthalmologist judges the correct acceptance of the lower segment by observing whether or not the child invariably raises the chin and depresses the eyes to look through the lower segment when small target material is presented at eye level or slightly above at a distance of 0.33 meter. The most satisfactory bifocal is a flat-top segment that traverses the entire width of the lens, eg, the executive bifocal. With this type of lens, regardless of the position in which the child depresses the eyes in straight downgaze, left and downgaze, or right and downgaze, the lower segment is simultaneously engaged by each eye. Care should be exercised by the parents to ensure that the glasses are in proper adjustment since tilted or crooked glasses result in one eye looking through the lower bifocal segment and the other eye looking above it. Some patients obviously need bifocals, and they are prescribed as the initial spectacles. For example, the child who, without glasses, has straight eyes for distance but 35Δ of esotropia for near and ±1.00 D cycloplegic refractive error needs bifocals. Substituting a miotic for bifocals when the patient needs glasses due to a refractive error usually does not succeed because the child tends to peer over the spectacles and abandons them. Miotics work best in lieu of glasses not in conjunction with glasses.

Two miotics have been used extensively in North America for accommodative esotropia, viz, isofluorophate (DFP) (Floropryl, 0.025% ointment) and echothiophate (PI) (Phospholine Iodide 0.125%). Isofluorophate is inactivated by water and must be dispensed either in *USP* anhydrous peanut oil or ophthalmic ointment. The strongest concentration that should be used for strabismus is 0.025%, and either one drop of liquid or a small bead of ointment is instilled in each eye daily. Echothiophate is stable in a water solution if it is refrigerated; the strongest concentration used for strabismus is 0.125%, with one drop being instilled in each eye each morning. Both drugs cause miosis, but more severe miosis is caused by DFP than by PI. Sustained miosis is often associated with pigmented hypertrophic irides ("cysts") at the pupillary border; these "cysts" jut out into the pupillary space and may seal the space shut if they are allowed to develop further by continuing the medication. This occurs more readily with DFP than with PI. After discontinuing the miotic, the "cysts" diminish in size but remain as an obvious pigmented hyperplastic mass on the pupillary border for years. The "cysts" can be prevented by instilling 2.5% phenylephrine hydrochloride twice daily; this slightly diminishes the miosis but does not interfere with the miotic function of potentiating the transmission of acetylcholine at the myoneural junction of the ciliary musculature. Miotics have a residual action for several days to a few weeks, making cycloplegia and mydriasis less than thorough during this period.

It is more difficult to work with DFP than with PI because of its propensity to be destroyed by water and the greater miosis it causes; however DFP performs better than PI in controlling the accommodative esodeviation. Echothiophate also has a systemic effect, ie, it destroys the cholinesterase in plasma and erythrocytes. This constitutes an additional risk for the patient undergoing anesthesia, particularly if other anticholinesterase drugs, eg, succinylcholine, are used during intubation to relax the pharyngeal muscles. As a result, the muscles used in respiration may be rendered functionless for a few hours, and the anesthesiologist may have to supply artificial ventilation for the patient until the muscles recover. Finally, subcapsular vacuoles, and even cataracts, have been reported in eyes receiving PI. Neither drug can be considered innocuous, and the indication for their use must be carefully evaluated. No patient should receive this medication without being observed at least every three months. After the patient's deviation is controlled, either the concentration may be halved or the frequency of instillation diminished progressively to every other day and then to every third day. The minimum dosage should control the deviation and allow fusion. The medication deteriorates with time, and the patient develops some degree of tolerance to it; these variables must also be considered. The medical approach to controlling accommodative esodeviation is more precarious and difficult to manage than the optic approach. Since accommodative esotropia requires long-term control, miotics are not the agents of choice for prolonged therapy. The prime importance of glasses in the management of accommodative esotropia has not been displaced by miotics.

The cause of accommodative esotropia determines the clinical course. Accommodative esotropia due to hypermetropia and a normal AC/A ratio remains well-controlled once glasses straighten the eyes. However, this is not true for accommodative esotropia due to a high AC/A ratio. Despite the use of glasses to immediately control the esotropia, there is a significant possibility that a gradual, nonaccommodative esotropia component will appear.

TABLE 12-2. Relationship Between the Deterioration Rate and the Severity of the High AC/A Ratio

Patients	AC/A	Deterioration Rate (%)
40	Normal	5
19	Slightly high	11
20	Moderately high	35
21	Severely high	43

Table 12-2 shows that the more severe the high AC/A ratio, the greater is the possibility of the patient deteriorating and developing nonaccommodative esotropia, thus escaping the control that glasses originally rendered (2).

Patients with a high AC/A ratio and a need for bifocals do not usually manifest improvement in the severity of their abnormal ratio until after 7 years of age. The hypermetropia disclosed by subsequent cycloplegic refraction usually increases until 6 years of age, levels off for two or more years, and after 8 years of age frequently decreases until the teens. Patients with accommodative esotropia controlled with glasses, including bifocals, are reexamined at six-month intervals until 6 years of age and annually thereafter.

Children who became constantly esotropic prior to receiving treatment and whose glasses have not reduced their angle to straight or children who were originally straight with glasses but escaped the control supplied by glasses and who are now esotropic with glasses require surgery for the quantity of esotropia measured at distance with their full corrective lens. Empirically, the author has learned that patients having a high AC/A ratio who require surgery should receive more than the customary amount of surgery done for that angle of esotropia. For example, if the angle of deviation would normally require 4-mm recession of the medial recti, the author would do a 5-mm bilateral medial rectus recession for the patient with a high AC/A ratio. Any child receiving surgery should have the amblyopia, if present, eliminated by the appropriate occlusion therapy prior to the surgery. If, after wearing glasses for one month, the eyes remain esotropic and there is no amblyopia, then surgery is performed. The author has not noticed improvement in the angle of esotropia in patients wearing glasses for several months. The constantly esotropic eyes either straighten promptly with glasses or assume an angle of esotropia that remains approximately the same until surgery is performed.

4 to 8 Years of Age

The treatment of accommodative esotropia in children between 4 and 8 years of age contrasts with that described for children under 4 years of age in that the minimum power lenses required to maintain fusion and provide maximum visual acuity can be determined and prescribed. With accommodative targets at distance and near and by doing the cover-uncover test, the least power plus lenses that keep the eyes straight are prescribed, including bifocals if necessary. Ideally, esophoria is demonstrable by an alternate cover test with these minimal plus lenses since it maintains a high degree of tone in the fusional divergence. This satisfies the objective of accommodative esotropia therapy, viz, reduce the esodeviation with an antiaccommodation measure just sufficiently to allow accommodative esophoria to replace accommodative esotropia. The object is not to convert accommodative esotropia to orthophoria. Maintaining orthophoria with glasses over several years, never putting a load on the patient's fusional divergence, decreases the probability of eventual withdrawal of glasses without symptoms of asthenopia, blurred vision, and diplopia. It is generally impossible to apply this objective of therapy for accommodative esotropia to children under 4 years of age because the examiner is unable to evoke a response in this age-group that is indicative of the visual acuity.

Over 8 Years of Age

In the treatment of accommodative esotropia in children 8 years of age and older, the ophthalmologist must realize that this is the earliest age at which improvement should be expected. The hypermetropia usually decreases, and the severity of the high AC/A ratio diminishes from this age into the early teens. The power of the spectacle plus lenses can usually be decreased and the bifocals reduced and frequently withdrawn. The prognosis for withdrawal of the spectacle must be related to the severity of the hypermetropia, the astigmatism, the anisometropia, and the AC/A ratio. Some patients who should have a good prognosis for part-time or full-time spectacle withdrawal but show no spontaneous improvement may be induced to remove their glasses after expanding their fusional vergence amplitude or at least encouraged to become more reliant on using their fusional divergence to its maximal potential. Patients are taught to limit their accommodation to that quantity that does not evoke more accommodative esodeviation than can be contained by the fusional divergence amplitude, even though the retinal image remains

blurred since less than adequate accommodation was applied to gain maximal visual acuity. This can be taught by either an orthoptist or an ophthalmologist by using diminishing strength miotics.

The orthoptist teaches dissociation exercises to enable the patient with accommodative esotropia to remove his glasses. First, the patient is taught to maintain straight eyes without glasses in the unaccommodative state, accepting blurred vision. Next, small increments of accommodation that are associated with increasing amounts of esophoria are allowed. Repeating this maneuver increases the fusional divergence amplitude. Gradually, larger amounts of esodeviation are withstood until, eventually, clear vision and straight eyes are maintained. Physiologic diplopia (framing) and bar reading (see chapter entitled Exodeviations) should be practiced during this routine to ensure against lapsing into esotropia with suppression and to guarantee maintenance of fusion with clear vision. Training to increase the fusional divergence amplitude may be done at the same time by using gradually stronger base-in prisms while watching television and reading or by employing stereoscopic or Polaroid vectographic techniques (Orthofusor).

By gradually diminishing the concentration or frequency of the instillation of the miotic, the fusional divergence may be expanded and possibly the glasses removed. The reduction of the dosage of either DFP or PI requires the patient to accommodate more in order to obtain clear vision. This causes greater esophoria which in turn puts more stress on the fusional divergence amplitude if binocularity is to be maintained. By gradually expanding the fusional divergence amplitude, some patients can eventually discontinue all medication, keeping the eyes straight and seeing well. The program ideally follows this plan:

1. Remove glasses and start 0.125% PI daily for one week.
2. Decrease to 0.06% PI daily for one week.
3. Decrease to 0.06% PI every other day for four doses.
4. Decrease to 0.06% PI every third day for three doses.
5. Decrease to 0.06% PI every fourth day for two doses.
6. Decrease to 0.06% PI every week for two doses.
7. Discontinue all medication.

The patient is examined each time the dosage is changed, and further decrease is not made unless the eyes are straight. This routine can be combined with orthoptic dissociation exercises and fusional divergence amplitude exercises.

These procedures are successful in patients 8 years of age or older with moderate refractive errors and in those with moderately severe high AC/A ratios. However, if the policy of providing no lens power above that necessary to keep the eyes straight is pursued from 4 years of age, then most of those who required medication or orthoptics to rid themselves of glasses at 8 years of age will have achieved the same result by 10 to 12 years of age.

NONACCOMMODATIVE ESODEVIATIONS

Nonaccommodative esodeviations are the various types of convergent strabismus not associated with accommodation. Whether or not the fusional vergences can control the esodeviation determines if the deviation is an esophoria or an esotropia.

The cause of nonaccommodative esodeviations is both neurogenic and anatomic. The innervating factor that causes convergence other than accommodative and fusional convergence is identified as tonic convergence. Accordingly, the innervational cause of nonaccommodative esotropia is reasoned to be some vague disturbance within the tonic vergences, resulting in either excessive tonic convergence or deficient tonic divergence. It is convenient, although unproved, to use this speculation to explain both congenital esotropia and the esotropia that gradually develops secondary to an anomaly that impairs the sight in one or both eyes of infants and young children.

The anatomic factors that probably account for some of the nonaccommodative esodeviation problems are primary anomalies, eg, abnormal medial recti, and secondary anomalies, eg, the change that occurs in the medial recti with excessive innervation, as encountered in deteriorated accommodative esotropia, abducens palsy, and Duane's syndrome.

CONGENITAL ESOTROPIA

Congenital esotropia is usually apparent to the parents shortly after the child's birth. After the first few days of life, when the eyes are open sufficiently for study, the esotropia is detected. Some parents claim the esotropia was not obvious until one or two months later but the esodeviation is open to subjective analysis, and it is difficult for the physician to procure good objective analysis.

Characteristically, the angle of convergence is large and constant, showing little sign of change with age in children without brain damage. A high percentage of brain-damaged infants have congenital esotropia but their angle of strabismus is usually more variable, frequently diminishing with age; occasionally, the esotropia is spontaneously replaced with exotropia between 6 months to 1 year of age.

Diagnosis

The majority of patients with congenital esotropia alternate fixation in the primary position and cross fixate on side gaze, using the right eye in left gaze and the left eye in right gaze, as illustrated in Figure 12-3. The minority who happen not to alternate their fixation have amblyopia in the nonpreferred eye which may be profound, as manifest by eccentric fixation. The cross-fixation pattern can be confusing and misleading to the examiner who is not experienced in examining infants with congenital esotropia. The examiner must learn that the absence of the abduction so frequently encountered in these infants is secondary to the cross-fixation habit. The infant who cross fixates has never abducted an eye, and the examiner finds it impossible to evoke an abduction response on either version or duction studies. The inexperienced examiner may assume that the patient has bilateral abducens paralysis. Similarly, the inexperienced examiner may mistakenly suspect unilateral abducens paralysis in the eccentrically fixating eye of a patient with a large angle of congenital esotropia who does not cross fixate and has amblyopia. To help avoid this pitfall, the examiner should be alert to this possibility and also realize that unilateral and bilateral congenital abducens paralysis are rare disorders; he should also be informed of the possibility of confusing abducens paralysis with Duane's syndrome and Möbius' syndrome.

Two diagnostic maneuvers can assist the examiner in differentiating congenital esotropia and its associated abduction limitation from abducens paralysis, Duane's syndrome, and Möbius' syndrome. By spinning the child with the head fixed in an upright position, clasped in the examiner's hands so it cannot be turned, and holding the child tightly against the examiner's chest, one swiftly accelerates and decelerates the patient's head horizontally through space. This labyrinthian stimulation, specifically of the horizontal semicircular canals, causes a subtle abducting movement of the eye on the side opposite to the direction of head acceleration that lasts for only a second. By closely concentrating on the eye, a favorably positioned second examiner can detect the abduction. A second method of producing abduction in the cross-fixating congenital esotrope is to occlude one eye for several days, and abduction will appear in the other eye.

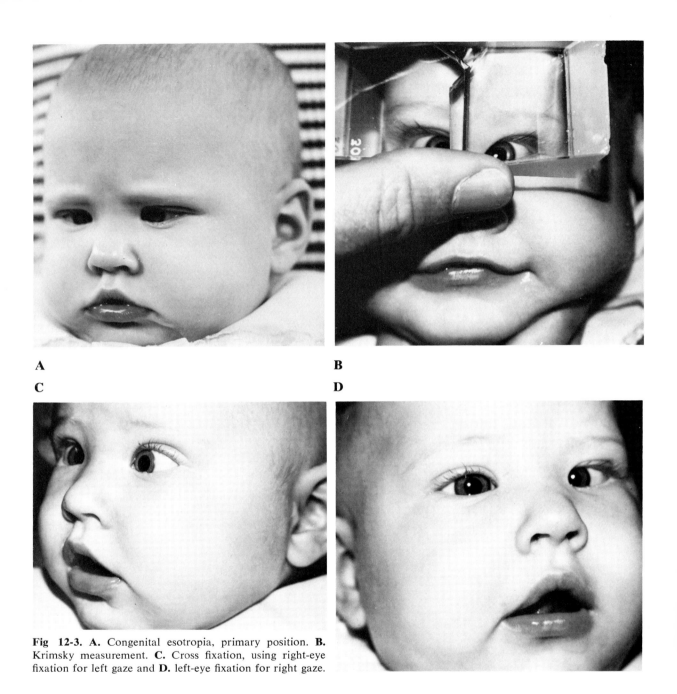

Fig 12-3. A. Congenital esotropia, primary position. **B.** Krimsky measurement. **C.** Cross fixation, using right-eye fixation for left gaze and **D.** left-eye fixation for right gaze.

The traction test performed in an anesthetized cross-fixating congenitally esotropic child, who manifests no abduction, is universally normal. No passive resistance to abduction is encountered. Also, with the patient under surgical plane anesthesia, the large angle of esotropia disappears, and often the eyes are divergent.

The esotropia angle is measured by the Krimsky prism technique in infants and young children (Fig 12-3, *B*) until the prism and alternate cover measurements are determinable. In infants and young children, usually only a horizontal deviation is present; however, the majority of children 2 to 3 years of age manifest a dissociated double hyperdeviation. Early surgical correction of the congenital esotropia does not reduce the incidence of this interesting cyclovertical disorder. The dissociated double hyperdeviation is manifest by the nonfixating eye being elevated and extorted. Alternate cover testing reveals that the eye behind the cover elevates and extorts, and the eye assuming fixation depresses and intorts, as illustrated in Figure 18-1, *A* and *B*. As the cover moves from eye to eye, this process repeats itself; this results in a positive vertical vergence with the cover before the right eye and a negative vertical vergence with the cover before the left eye, with simultaneous movements being dextrocycloversion with the cover before the right eye and levocycloversion with the cover before the left eye. The fact that these cyclovertical movements occur simultaneously with the bilateral abducting movements during the alternate cover testing in a congenital esotrope makes them difficult to detect. However, they are easily detected after the horizontal deviation is eliminated by surgery. The presence of dissociated double hyperdeviation is not pathognomonic for congenital esotropia, although the majority of congenital esotropes have it. Dissociated double hyperdeviation is infrequently encountered in patients with exotropia and in patients having horizontally straight eyes.

Version studies in infants under 1 year of age are usually normal, but overacting inferior obliques appear in the majority of the older congenitally esotropic children. This problem also occurs with the same incidence, regardless of whether or not early surgery was performed and the horizontal deviation eliminated.

The cycloplegic refraction can be anything, but it is usually equal in the two eyes and hypermetropic by the usual amount for the chronologic age.

In older children in whom sensory testing is reliable, the absence of binocular vision is the invariable finding in a patient who has received no treatment to straighten the congenitally esotropic eyes. Children who are straight as a result of early surgery often manifest peripheral fusion with NRC, but they never have central fusion. Children who were straightened at a young age and then either had a return of esotropia or developed secondary exotropia may have suppression and ARC.

Management

The management of congenital esotropia essentially involves surgical straightening of the eyes. The controversial aspects of this need are when and how the surgery is best accomplished. The need for eliminating amblyopia, if present, prior to surgery is not controversial. Alternate occlusion therapy may benefit the minority of patients having a propensity for amblyopia until the surgery is performed, but it is of no other value. Alternate occlusion therapy for congenitally esotropic patients to prevent suppression and ARC is completely unfounded. Suppression and ARC are adaptations to NRC fusion; they never develop unless binocular vision, which is lacking in congenitally deviated eyes, is already present. Apparently, a requisite for the conditioned reflex of single binocular vision development is straight eyes or eyes at least within 10Δ of being horizontally straight during infancy or early childhood. Therefore, treating congenital esotropia with alternate occlusion for a few years, until the child is sufficiently mature to be taught by orthoptics how to fuse, and then performing the necessary surgery illustrates a gross lack of knowledge about the disorder.

The best single binocular vision obtainable is peripheral single binocular vision. However, this is important since the fusional vergence amplitudes are normal with peripheral fusion, and it is this attribute that maintains straight eyes for these patients for the remainder of their lives. The patient who obtains only cosmetic improvement with surgery and no peripheral fusion eventually suffers a gradual deviation of the eyes with increasing age; this usually is a secondary exotropia. Also, because of the high incidence of associated dissociative double hypertropia, the nonfixating eye tends to be cosmetically upturned. Although secondary surgery can benefit these cosmetic horizontal and vertical problems, the improvement is not permanent and eventually the deviation returns. This future hardship is prevented by acquiring peripheral fusion for the congenitally esotropic patient, and the benefit of gross stereopsis is also provided.

The statistics regarding results of fusion in patients with congenital esotropia are difficult to obtain; however, some factors essential for binocular vision can be identified. Single binocular vision is not forthcoming unless the deviation is reduced to 10Δ or less. Secondly, fusion is not obtained in children who first achieve this alignment after 4 years of age. Thirdly, the percentage of patients obtaining fusion after surgical elimination of their deviation seems to be greater in those whose eyes were straightened before 1 year of age than in older children. Obtaining data to support the above statements is more difficult than one might think due to problems associated with accumulating absolute case material to show that there was definitely constant congenital esotropia without previous opportunity for fusion development and because results of surgery in various age-groups must be investigated. Parents' uncertainty that the esotropia was constant rather than intermittent and the possibility that the strabismus was actually acquired after single binocular vision was developed create problems in investigating this issue. Furthermore, pseudostrabismus created by the wide, flat infantile nose, small interpupillary distance, and epicanthi cause many parents to assume that esotropia is present when actually the eyes are straight. Then, if a real esotropia gradually begins, due to the pseudoesotropia existing previously, the parents are inclined to think that the esotropia has been present since birth.

Surgery is performed ideally at 6 months of age in children having no brain damage. By this age, the examiner can assess the Krimsky prism measurement of the esotropia angle and the patient's fixation ability. All children are refracted, and their fundi are viewed prior to committing the child to surgery. Amblyopia is overcome, if present, with occlusion therapy prior to surgery. Assuming that good pediatric anesthesiology is available and that the surgeon is a knowledgeable technician in dealing with extraocular muscles, early surgery for congenital esotropia is safe and rewarding. Routinely, the medial recti are recessed maximally (5 mm), presuming the angle of esotropia is 40∆ or more. Patients with residual esotropia angles of 15∆ or more at six weeks postoperatively receive secondary surgery on the lateral recti, ie, resection from 5 to 8 mm, according to the magnitude of the angle. The surgical objective in children under 4 years of age is to place the eyes within 10∆ of orthophoria, not simply to reduce the angle of esotropia. The response to surgery in terms of the quantity of improvement in the angle of esotropia is variable in infants; therefore, it is justifiable to operate on only two muscles and assess the result. Following this scheme, patients with esotropia angles up to 70∆ have approximately a 50 percent chance of requiring only one operation, whereas those with angles greater than 70∆ have a greater chance of needing the second procedure. For this reason, in infants with large angles of esotropia, some surgeons prefer to operate on more than two muscles immediately. Also, some surgeons routinely recess and resect the horizontal recti of one eye, rather than doing bimedial recessions; they claim similarly good results. It is folly to claim one approach to be better than another since each surgeon has developed confidence in his own surgical method, and this individual technique should be followed. The important issue is to do something surgically to straighten the eyes; ideally, this should be performed when the patient is young. If the surgeon performs a recession-resection on the horizontal recti of one eye and a residual esotropia persists at six weeks postoperatively, then a re-

cession-resection quantitated to the angle of deviation should be performed on the other eye. A guide to the quantity of surgery performed for various esotropic angles is listed in Table 12-3. To read from top down is for recession of the medial recti of both eyes (MROU) and resection of the lateral recti of both eyes (LROU). To read from bottom up is for recession of the medial rectus (MR) and resection of the lateral rectus (LR) of one eye. These quantities of surgery are not varied according to the age of the patient. Children 4 years of age or younger receive surgery simultaneously on only two horizontal recti, but older children may have surgery simultaneously on as many as four horizontal recti if the angle of deviation is sufficiently large to require it. Table 12-3 is applicable to both primary and secondary surgery. Coexisting A or V patterns are also corrected by vertically displacing the horizontal recti at the same time they are recessed or resected. Overacting inferior obliques are also corrected by recessing them if they are coexistent with the esotropia.

The surgical objective in children under 4 years of age is to reduce the congenital esotropia to within 10∆ of straight, but in older children the objective is to undercorrect the total angle by approximately 15∆. The surgeon wishes to give the young child an opportunity to develop single binocular vision, and straight or nearly straight eyes are a requisite for this; however, cosmetic improvement is the only objective in older children. The patient who does not develop single binocular vision usually deviates spontaneously into exotropia within several years after surgery, and having a residual of 15∆ esotropia delays this unfortunate sequel. The fear of postoperative drift into exotropia 10 to 30 years after surgery is no reason to deny cosmetic surgery to the patient who has no chance of obtaining single binocular vision because the secondary exotropia can always be eliminated by secondary surgery. Single binocular vision is the benefit given to congenitally esotropic infants

TABLE 12-3. Quantity of Surgery for Various Esotropic Angles

ET	Recess MROU	Resect LROU
15∆	3 mm	4 mm
20∆	3.5 mm	5 mm
25∆	4 mm	6 mm
30∆	4.5 mm	7 mm
35∆	5 mm	8 mm
ET	Recess MR and	Resect LR

by early surgery since this result ensures straight eyes for the remainder of their lives, except for the possibility that accommodative esotropia may develop later and glasses may be required to control it.

Accommodative esotropia and amblyopia both occur frequently in youngsters after the congenital esotropia is eliminated by surgery, and single binocular peripheral fusion is present. Therefore, the patient must be closely followed during the first 5 years of life, and appropriate treatment for each of these disorders must be promptly instituted.

Dissociated double hyperdeviation often creates a cosmetic problem for these patients. Surgical elimination of the esotropia does not alter the hyperdeviation. The patient who achieves fusion has the advantage over the patient who does not since the upturning of the nonfixating eye is kept latent. Even such a relatively ideal result as dissociated double hyperphoria may lapse with visual inattention or fatigue into dissociated double hypertrophia; if the hyperdeviation is large, it is cosmetically disfiguring. However, the patient who has no fusion ability has a constantly upturned eye that alternates with the other if alternate fixation is present. The dissociated double hypertropia occurs in all degrees of severity and often is sufficiently disfiguring to require cosmetic improvement. The surgery that offers the best improvement for this difficult problem is resection of the inferior recti. Recessions of the superior recti and inferior obliques render minimal change in the upturning of these eyes. The quantity of upturning may vary in the right and left eyes; however, except in the patient who has marked dissociative hypertropia in one eye and minimal upturning in the other eye, both inferior recti should be resected (see chapter entitled Dissociated Hyperdeviations).

The older patient with congenital esotropia, without binocular vision and with good vision in each eye, who sees only the Bagolini streak presented to the fixating eye, does not experience diplopia after surgery. Therefore, the possibility of postoperative diplopia should never be mentioned to the patient preoperatively. This contrasts with the patient having acquired esotropia and abnormal retinal correspondence who always experiences diplopia for a variable period of time after surgery.

ESOTROPIA ASSOCIATED WITH IMPAIRED SIGHT

An anomaly that either prevents development of sight in an infant or appears in a young child after the sight has developed is usually associated with an esotropia that is first apparent at 6 months of age or six months after the anomaly was acquired. The esotropia gradually increases but usually does not increase to equal the large angle so frequently found in patients with congenital esotropia.

The fixation is irretrievably ruined in the involved eye, and, consequently, the angle of deviation cannot be measured with prism and alternate cover techniques. The angle must be estimated by the Krimsky prism reflex test. Either a high or low AC/A ratio may cause the near deviation to be greater than or less than the distant deviation. Also, the poorly sighted eye often gradually develops an associated hypertropia in addition to the esotropia, and this is frequently associated with an overacting inferior oblique muscle.

Ophthalmoscopy provides the answer regarding the cause of this disorder in many patients. If there is retinoblastoma involvement of the macula, strabismus may be the presenting feature of this serious disease (Fig 12-4). Therefore, every strabismic patient should receive an examination of the fundi as soon as possible.

Presuming the visual anomaly is uncorrectable, surgical elimination of the esotropia is for cosmetic improvement. Surgery can be performed at any age the parents wish, but they should be urged to have the surgery performed before the child is 4 years old. Children become sensitive about their appearance by this age, and every effort should be made to prevent any psychologic trauma resulting from this strabismus before it can become an issue.

The objective of the surgery is to undercorrect the angle of esotropia by 15Δ because of the tendency for eventual replacement of the esotropia with secondary exotropia. If the exotropia becomes obvious during the ensuing years, the initial surgery

Fig 12-4. Retinoblastoma as a cause of esotropia associated with impaired sight.

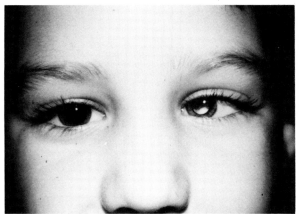

can be reversed. The parents of the esotropic youngster should be informed of the tendency for the eyes to drift outward as the child matures; they should also be assured that the probable secondary exotropia can be managed surgically when and if necessary in the future, as well as the primary esotropic cosmetic defect that confronts them at present.

A recession-resection procedure on the horizontal rectus muscle of the involved eye is the usual technique employed to correct the esotropia. Recessions of the medial recti may also be used if the surgeon chooses to do so, but the parents usually manifest uneasiness over the issue of surgery being performed on the good eye. Although there is no medical foundation for the worry, the emotional trauma endured by most parents and/or patients over this issue, despite explanation and assurance by the surgeon regarding the safety and good prognosis for correction of the esotropic angle by doing symmetric surgery on each eye, results in most surgeons resigning themselves to routinely performing the surgery on only the involved eye. If the inferior oblique muscle of the involved eye is overactive, it is recessed at the same time the horizontal recti are recessed. If hypertropia of the involved eye is apparent in both right and left gaze, and the traction test with the patient under anesthesia reveals no resistance to passive infraduction, then resection of the inferior rectus muscle is added to the surgery performed on the horizontal recti and inferior obliques. If the traction test reveals positive resistance to passive infraduction the superior rectus muscle is recessed instead of resecting the inferior rectus muscle. The traction test should be re-evaluated at least after the superior rectus muscle has been disinserted to determine if the test has been converted to normal before proceeding with the recession of this muscle. The surgeon should never attempt to solve the esotropia and hypertropia by operating on all four recti muscles, since this would expose the eye to vascular embarrassment of the anterior segment.

Undercorrection resulting from the surgery can be approached secondarily by converting less than maximal recession of the medial rectus and resection of the lateral rectus to the maximal amounts of 5 mm and 8 mm, respectively. Provided maximal recession-resection was initially performed and a cosmetic esotropia defect persists six months postoperatively, a Z lengthening procedure can be performed on the medial rectus muscle, along with a repeat resection of the lateral rectus muscle. No quantity of surgery can be stated for the re-resection. The lateral rectus muscle must be investigated for its tautness, and by overlapping the muscle while it is still in the resection clamp to the eye placed in the primary position, the surgeon can determine the resection quantity required to reattach the lateral rectus muscle to its scleral insertion site.

Overcorrection is more easily managed surgically than undercorrection since the surgeon performing the secondary procedure simply reverses the primary surgery partially or entirely, depending on the preoperative and postoperative measurements. There is no reason to delay management of obvious postoperative overcorrection more than two or three months because the secondary exotropia continues to increase. If hypermetropic spectacles were required for the good eye, the plus power is reduced or withdrawn as soon as overcorrection is apparent in children. However, any benefit produced by this method is usually short-lived, as the inevitable exo drift continues. Prescribing minus lens spectacles for the patient with no significant refractive error with the hope of reversing the overcorrection is no more successful than reducing the plus lens spectacles worn preoperatively.

Prior to doing primary surgery, the accommodative esotropia component must be considered. This demands either plus spectacles or miotic trial if the refractive error of the fixating eye exceeds +1.50 D. Also, only the distance esotropia is treated surgically. For the patient with a high AC/A ratio and greater near than distance esotropia, a miotic is required if only the near esotropia is cosmetically disfiguring. Surgery can never be performed in this instance without producing exotropia for distance. If plus lenses maintain a satisfactory cosmetic alignment, the surgeon who substitutes surgery for glasses more often renders a disservice to the patient rather than a benefit because secondary exotropia occurs, usually soon postoperatively. Contact lenses substituted for the plus spectacles would have been a more prudent method of removing the spectacles than surgery.

DIVERGENCE PARALYSIS

Strabismus due to the accommodative convergence reflex or the tonic convergence reflex is so prevalent that the examiner may overlook the possibility that a concomitant esodeviation is due to any other cause. Consequently, divergence paralysis can easily remain unrecognized.

The abrupt onset of an acquired concomitant esodeviation, maximal for distance fixation which diminishes to orthophoria at a near fixation point of 1 meter or less, that remains relatively unchanged in lateral gaze is divergence paralysis (3–5). The onset of this disorder may be at any age; the first symptom is homonymous diplopia for distant objects. Despite the esotropia in the primary position, either eye abducts in response to lateral version testing. The fusional divergence amplitude may be diminished or absent, although there is controversy regarding this finding (6). Some patients with divergence paralysis also have an associated convergence weakness with heteronymous diplopia and exodeviation for fixation points within 0.5 to 0.33 meter.

Etiologic factors are multiple, often obscure, and frequently associated with known or suspected intracranial disease. Divergence paralysis may occur with increased intracranial pressure (7), head trauma (8), encephalitis, tabes dorsalis, multiple sclerosis, tumors and cysts of the cerebellum, acoustic neuroma, astrocytoma of the parietal lobe, glioma of the pons, vascular accidents, and in the resolving stage of Foville's syndrome. Divergence paralysis may disappear or improve after the primary cause has been eliminated.

Jampolsky (6) makes a plea for more accurate diagnosis of divergence paralysis; he claims that it is frequently confused with late onset esotropia and bilateral palsy of the sixth cranial nerve. He correctly criticizes the diagnosis unless it can be proven that there is total absence of divergence amplitude and that abduction of each eye is normal. He contends that bilateral palsy of the sixth cranial nerve may result from the lesion in the floor of the fourth ventricle; this lesion also affects the medial longitudinal fasciculi, reducing the adduction in each eye as manifest by version stimulation but leaving the convergence power intact. With only partial involvement of the sixth cranial nerve and medial longitudinal fasciculi, some abduction and adduction of each eye in response to horizontal version testing could conceivably simulate divergence palsy. However, it would be suspected that such a patient would manifest nystagmoid horizontal excursions of each eye on attempted dextroversion and levoversion. Despite one's best efforts, the diagnosis of divergence paralysis is usually equivocal, and as the clinical course of this motility disorder is followed, frequently the diagnosis must be changed to bilateral palsy of the sixth cranial nerve. However, the important issue is that the diagnosis of divergence palsy, whether it be a secure or an equivocal one, demands careful and prolonged neurophthalmologic study.

Treatment of divergence paralysis is palliative, seeking only to relieve the diplopia with occlusion therapy or prisms, until the neurophthalmologic status has solidified. If the paralysis persists for six months without change, then recession of the medial recti is justified and provides a good prognosis for success.

REFERENCES

1. Parks MM: Abnormal accommodative convergence in squint. Arch Ophthalmol 59:364, 1958
2. Manley DE, Parks MM: To be published
3. Walsh FF, Hoyt WF: Clinical Neuro-Ophthalmology, ed. 3. Baltimore: Williams & Wilkins, 1969
4. Burian HM: New Orleans Symposium on Strabismus. St. Louis: Mosby, 1971, 231–232
5. Cunningham RD: Divergence paralysis. Am J Ophthalmol 74:630, 1972
6. Jampolsky A: Ocular divergence mechanisms. Trans Am Ophthalmol Soc 68:748, 1970
7. Kirkham TH, Bird AC, Sanders MD: Divergence paralysis with raised intracranial pressure. Br J Ophthalmol 56:776, 1972
8. Rutkowski, PC, Burian HM: Divergence paralysis following head trauma. Am J Ophthalmol 73:660, 1972

13

Concomitant Exodeviations

Visual axes that form a divergent angle as they proceed outward comprise an exodeviation. Diverged visual axes kept latent by single binocular vision constitute exophoria, but when manifest, the misaligned visual axes constitute exotropia. Many patients with divergent deviations vacillate between phoria and tropia; this fluctuating condition is designated as intermittent exotropia.

ETIOLOGY

A disturbance in the tonic horizontal vergence is usually considered the cause of most primary divergent deviations. However, since so little is known about the total spectrum of vergence innervations that disjugately drive the eyes, other than accommodative convergence and fusional vergence, such speculation is rather meaningless. There appears to be some disruption in the usual balance of tonic vergence innervations; this results in either a deficiency of convergence innervation or an excess of divergence innervation. Whatever the cause of such innervational disruption, it seems to be genetically influenced because the hereditary aspects of the primary divergent deviation are inescapably obvious to the ophthalmologist.

Secondary anatomic factors probably occur within and surrounding the extraocular muscles; they account for a gradual increase in the divergent angle in both the intermittently and constantly exotropic patients. Excess innervation to the lateral recti possibly results in their hypertrophy; also, in long-standing constant exotropia, the elastic fibers surrounding the fascial and conjunctival tissues may add their force to the divergent pull of the visual axes, further increasing the exotropic angle. There-

fore, it may be difficult to determine which part of the cause is primarily innervational and which is secondarily anatomic. The interplay of innervational and anatomic forces is displayed in the patient who sustains a traumatic unilateral cataract. Although the eyes were orthophoric prior to the injury, within a few weeks following the disruption of binocular vision by the acquired lens opacity, the injured eye usually begins to diverge in adults and in children over 5 years of age. In younger children the injured eye usually converges. Over the years the divergent injured eye becomes increasingly exotropic, and, eventually, the traction test reveals resistance to passive adduction and shortening of the temporal conjunctiva and Tenon's capsule extending between the temporal limbus and the outer canthus. Apparently, when ungoverned by binocular vision, tonic divergence prevails over tonic convergence, and, eventually, the original innervational alteration is secondarily reinforced by anatomic changes in the extraocular muscles and surrounding tissues.

Anatomic causes of exotropia may be the primary factor in rather than the consequence of prior innervational imbalance to the extraocular muscles. Surgical overcorrections of esotropia, trauma to the orbit causing either a palsy of the medial rectus or an adhesive cicatricial pull on the temporal aspect of the globe, or osteologic disorders of the face and cranium, eg, the shallow diverged orbits in Crouzon's disease, are examples of anatomic abnormalities that produce exotropia.

CLINICAL CHARACTERISTICS

EXOPHORIA

Small amounts of exophoria in adults and even relatively large amounts in youngsters are usually asymptomatic. Discomfort or visual disturbances are symptoms of exophoria. The discomfort is manifest by vague asthenopia, which gradually increases during prolonged detailed visual tasks and dissipates with rest. The visual symptoms are momentary diplopia vacillating with momentary blurred vision. Symptoms occur when the fatigue threshold of fusional convergence is exceeded. As the patient finds it more difficult to maintain fusional convergence, he may substitute accommodative convergence which is necessarily associated with accommodation. Visual detail is blurred during purposeless application of accommodation. As the accommodation is relaxed, allowing the vision to clear, the accommodative convergence which was substituted for the exhausted fusional convergence is also decreased. The latent divergent deviation becomes manifest, and while it persists there is heteronymous diplopia. The response to the diplopia stimulus is to again apply the synkinetic near reflex, ie, overaccommodation and convergence, thus blurring the vision and eliminating the diplopia. Repeating this cycle creates the symptoms of momentary blurred vision vacillating with mometary diplopia.

The symptoms of exophoria occur for distant visual tasks if the exodeviation angle is significant for distance viewing and insignificant for near and vice versa for the opposite distance-near exodeviation measurements. Convergent insufficiency, manifest by a greater near than distance exodeviation, is more prevalent and accounts for the bulk of symptomatic exophoria. Students in the upper grades of school and adults involved in pursuing prolonged near visual tasks can be troubled by the recurrence of these symptoms. Many exophoric patients can anticipate the onset of their symptoms after having read either for a certain number of minutes or a certain number of pages of text. They usually describe the symptoms of "burning and watering eyes," followed soon thereafter with the "doubling and blurring" of the print if they attempt to persevere with the reading. Most exophoric patients learn to solve the latter symptoms, granted they continue reading, by closing or covering one eye. This is followed by a soporific state which they describe as "sleepiness," and the reading assignment they attempted is interrupted by sleep or the distraction of daydreaming. Poor health and chronic fatigue hasten the onset of the symptoms after the visual tasks are started. The exophoric symptoms probably play a greater role in subtly determining the patient's vocation than he is aware; they impose a significant hardship on the patient's genuine intent and desire to successfully complete a competitive academic program.

INTERMITTENT EXOTROPIA

Intermittent exotropia is usually a divergent deviation having its onset during infancy or early childhood. It may be noted as early as during the first few months of life. The parents are often convinced of the repeated outward turning of one or both of the infant's eyes by the sixth month. Yet, in some children, it may never be noticed until a much later age, eg, the seventh or eighth year of life. All but a small percentage of the total number of cases are manifest during the early years of childhood. Once the intermittent exotropia is manifest, it either remains unchanged or gradually deteriorates to a constant exotropia; it only rarely undergoes partial disappearance. There are some documented cases of patients who manifested intermittent exotropia

during early childhood and then without receiving treatment converted to exophoria in late childhood; they seemed to continue to be asymptomatic during their early adulthood. Possibly these patients are those who supposedly have the onset of intermittent exotropia in adulthood. The clinical course of the intermittent exotropia is difficult to document in those few patients who apparently improve spontaneously with growth because of their fading memory associated with increasing age and the extremely varied attitude patients have toward the visual and cosmetic aspects associated with this disorder. Disregarding the patients' statements and ignoring the matter of relative frequency of phoria and tropia, if the alternate cover measurements of the exodeviation were plotted over the patient's lifetime, probably only rarely would the patient show a significant permanent reduction in the exoangle with increasing age. Essentially, the exoangle is primarily a motor innervational disorder established during infancy and kept latent in the majority of the afflicted individuals most of the time by the sensory-motor innervation of binocular vision. The interplay of the motor etiology and the sensory-motor compensation allows for a spectrum of possible clinical manifestations of intermittent exotropia. Once the tropic aspect of this divergent deviation occurs, it usually recurs according to a pattern peculiar to each patient throughout the remainder of his life. The pattern of recurrence of the exotropia that varies widely is the principal feature distinguishing one case from another.

The tropic phase of intermittent exotropia is aggravated by many factors. Since binocular vision is the essential compensatory sensory-motor factor, the patient must be visually alert to his environment and willing to make the effort to maintain binocular vision. Daydreaming, visual distraction induced by thinking and speaking, fatigue, illness, and drowsiness present immediately after awakening are the usual factors that cause exotropia to replace exophoria. Distance viewing rather than near viewing is frequently more productive of exotropia. In some patients, exposure to bright illumination, eg, sunlight, is a striking aggravating factor; when exotropia occurs, this exposure causes sufficient annoyance to precipitate the immediate reflex closure of one eye. The unilateral contraction of the orbicularis may be so obvious that the parent presents the child to the ophthalmologist for this reason and is unaware of a divergent deviation.

The tropic phase tends to increase in many of the affected patients, possibly even the majority. The increase is by way of changes in frequency and duration. Instead of the tropia occurring only once or twice per day as it originally did, it tends to recur many times per day with increasing age; it also tends to remain for many minutes, instead of the original momentary duration. Eventually, in some patients the increased recurrence and duration of tropia seem to almost merge into a continuous exotropia. In patients whose sensory-motor compensation for the divergent deviation deteriorates to this extent, the last stage of their intermittent exotropia is usually characterized by retention of the phoric phase only for near seeing; they are constantly exotropic for distance viewing. Yet, other patients tend to retain the same frequency and duration of intermittent exotrophia for years; occasionally, they have exacerbations and remissions of the tropic phase related to the general health, the state of rest, and various disturbances that may occur in the daily routine. Finally, a few patients may manifest the tropic phase intermittently for several months to years when they are young and then improve spontaneously for several months to years, becoming constantly exophoric and never exotropic. Some of these patients suffer recurrences of the exotropia when they are older, but probably others do not. Most of these latter patients eventually become lost to follow-up, and their phoria-tropia status in later life remains unknown.

EXOTROPIA

The clinical characteristics of constant exotropia are determined by its cause. Constant exotropia is the result of several possible causes, eg, deteriorated intermittent exotropia, a poor seeing or blind eye. In congenital constant exotropia, binocular vision has never had an opportunity to develop, and the misaligned eyes constantly manifest abnormal motor innervation to the extraocular muscles. This is a rare disorder compared to congenital esotropia, but the author has documented its existence in six infants under 6 months of age.

Congenital esotropia may indirectly become the cause of constant exotropia since the absence of the ability to develop binocular vision is characteristic of congenital esotropes, unless the eyes were straightened by surgery while the patient was still young. The congenital esotrope soon becomes too old to initiate the cortical neurophysiologic pathways required by binocular vision, even though surgery has straightened the eyes. Although the eyes may appear well-aligned for a few years after surgery, an increasing exotropia gradually evolves in those without binocular vision, despite normal visual acuity in each eye. Also, some congenitally esotropic patients gradually change to exotropia without surgery; this trend is prevalent among children with cerebral palsy.

OBJECTIVE SIGNS

The accommodative convergence to accommodation (AC/A) ratio determines the difference between the exodeviation measured at distance and at near fixation. Patients with exodeviations that measure similarly at 6 meters and 0.33 meter while the examiner controls the patient's accommodation have a normal AC/A ratio. Greater deviations at distance or at near are the product of an abnormal AC/A ratio; the high AC/A ratio causes greater exodeviation at distance, and the low AC/A ratio causes greater exodeviation at near. According to Duane's classification, exodeviation greater at distance is divergence excess; exodeviation greater at near is convergence insufficiency. Common usage of Duane's classification during the past 70 years has served the clinician well by separating the exodeviation into three categories; the third category is exodeviation with neither divergence excess nor convergence insufficiency since the exodeviation is the same for distance and near. Variations in these three categories of deviation are found in all exodeviations, regardless of whether it is constant exophoria, intermittent exotropia, or constant exotropia.

EXOPHORIA

Exophoria is a latent deviation with good fusional vergence amplitude and no amblyopia. Bifixation is maintained despite the phoria, and normal stereoacuity proves its existence.

INTERMITTENT EXOTROPIA

Intermittent exotropia is also associated with normal fusional vergence amplitudes and no amblyopia. In exophoric patients, the fusional vergence amplitudes are used to maintain bifixation; this is sufficient to prevent amblyopia. The stereoacuity is almost always normal when the patient is phoric, but there is no stereopsis when the patient is exotropic.

Young patients quickly adapt sensorially to the exotropic phase by developing suppression and anomalous retinal correspondence (ARC), thus freeing themselves of diplopia and visual confusion. The suppression scotoma projecting into space soon becomes large, and the involved temporal retina extends from the hemiretinal line to beyond the locus where the object of regard is projected as an image (Fig 8-4). Profound as the sensorial adaptations become, the moment the eyes converge to straight, normal retinal correspondence occurs, with bifixation functioning at a peak level. To gain the advantage of stereopsis, visual alertness and willingness to make the effort to attain this visual reward are required. With inattention or a reduction in the desire for maintaining stereoscopic viewing, the effort to keep the eyes straight is terminated and the moment exotropia ensues, suppression and ARC viewing replace the stereoscopic view. Children 10 years of age and older who have not developed the sensorial adaptations when the eyes diverge are beyond the age at which they can develop them. Hence, they experience persistent heteronymous diplopia while the exotropia prevails. Although the diplopia is annoying, perhaps it is more acceptable than the asthenopia produced by struggling to keep the eyes straight when fatigued. However, these patients experience vexing symptoms while they are exotropic during certain visual circumstances, eg, while driving, the road seems to split into two roads and the oncoming automobile headlights become diplopic. The intermittent exotropic patient who has instantaneous suppression and ARC while tropic is much less annoyed visually than his counterpart who is devoid of these sensorial adaptations.

Measurements of the exodeviation while the distance and near accommodation are controlled are essential data best obtained by the cover test, using prisms to quantitate the exoangle. A muscle light should not be used as a fixating target for either distance or near accommodation because the exotropic patient frequently overaccommodates subconsciously, using the extra accommodative convergence to reduce the exoangle. The blurred image of the muscle light offers no deterrence to this method of compensating for the divergent deviation; however, the images of small symbols that are fixated demand an accurate accommodative response in order to be identified allowing the examiner to obtain valid measurements of the total exoangle. The exodeviation may also vary in upgaze and downgaze (A or V pattern) and in right and left gaze from the primary position just as the distance and near measurements may vary. These various gaze positions are recorded for distance viewing, plus the straight ahead near position. Versions often reveal inferior and/or superior oblique muscle dysfunction, and this should always be recorded. Long-standing exodeviations have a relatively great percentage of associated oblique muscle dysfunctions, and, since A and V patterns are frequently associated with the oblique muscle dysfunctions, long-standing intermittent exotropic patients have an increased incidence of A and V patterns.

A high AC/A ratio is more frequently encountered in intermittent exotropia than a low AC/A ratio, and younger intermittent exotropic children tend to have a more significantly high AC/A ratio than older children. Exodeviations measuring 20Δ to 35Δ at distance and 5Δ to 10Δ at near are common in young children, but with increasing age the near measurement tends to increase, causing the distance and near deviation to approximate each other. Viewing the near accommodative target through +3.00 lenses increases the near exodeviation measurement in most patients, regardless of the nature of the AC/A ratio; those with a high AC/A ratio experience the greatest effect. However, the near prism and alternate cover measurement obtained through +3.00 lenses has not provided more helpful information for the management of exodeviation than simply the distance and near accommodation controlled prism and alternate cover measurements. Some authors (1) have a different opinion and use the +3.00 lens near prism and alternate cover measurement to determine the muscles for surgical correction of the exodeviation. Their reasoning is based on the dual premise that (1) a central nervous system center controls the divergence, and (2) divergence innervation flows from this center when looking at distance and ceases when fixating at near. Therefore, an excess of divergence innervation would cause greater exodeviation at distance than at near. They also assume that the lateral recti are the diverging muscles and the medial recti are the converging muscles; from this, they deduct that the diverging muscles should be weakened in patients with an excess of divergence. From these premises they reason that patients with similar distance and near exodeviation measurements possess some unknown factor affecting the extraocular muscles and surrounding fascia, causing the divergence of the visual axes; whatever this factor, the exodeviation does not result from excessive innervational flow from the divergence center to the lateral recti. They call this basic exodeviation since excessive contraction of the lateral recti is not considered to be the primary cause of basic exodeviation. They advise recession of the lateral rectus muscle and resection of the medial rectus muscle of the same eye, presuming that this surgery produces a similar effect on straightening the diverged visual axes for both distance and near. They also reason that the innervational dispatch of the convergence center to the medial recti is deficient in patients with convergence insufficiency; they advise resection of the medial recti for this disorder. If one subscribes to the above reasoning, then prism and alternate cover near measurements through +3.00 lenses can provide some changes that make a particular case difficult to classify. For example, a patient's divergence excess measurements may be converted with the +3.00 lenses to basic exodeviation measurements, consequently, this patient is reclassified as having pseudodivergence excess. Other patients initially classified as having basic exodeviation will be changed by the +3.00 lenses to have convergence insufficiency measurements, and presumably they are reclassified as having pseudobasic exodeviation. Patients with convergence insufficiency cannot have their initial diagnosis changed by the +3.00 lenses; the only possible change is an increased exodeviation measurement at near.

Two weaknesses in the above reasoning create unnecessary confusion. The first is the assumption that a patient having greater exodeviation at distance than at near (divergence excess) is etiologically unrelated to another patient having similar distance and near exodeviation (basic exodeviation). It is relatively more appealing to theorize that the distance exodeviation in all patients is solely due to disturbance in the balance of opposing tonic horizontal vergence innervations, regardless of whether the near exodeviation is identical to, greater than, or less than the distance exodeviation. Congenital esotropia is theorized to result from the opposite disturbance in tonic horizontal vergences, and no consideration is given to whether the near esotropia is identical or dissimilar to the distance esotropia. The second weakness in the reasoning in the preceding paragraph is the reluctance to use the synkinetic near reflex to explain the differences in the distance-near exodeviation measurements; a normal AC/A ratio causes similar distance and near measurements, a high AC/A ratio causes greater distance exodeviation, and a low AC/A ratio causes greater near exodeviation. The AC/A ratio is used to explain differences in distance-near esodeviation measurements; therefore, the author believes it should also be used to explain the differences in distance-near exodeviation measurements. These two weaknesses are overcome by assuming that the interplay between the tonic vergence disturbance and the AC/A ratio explains all possible distance-near measurements encountered in the exodeviations. Therefore, no case need be classified as "pseudo" something because of a near measurement obtained with +3.00 D spheres.

Youngsters with divergent deviations tend to reveal less exodeviation at near than at distance by the prism and alternate cover test. This suggests that their AC/A ratio is pliable to the extent that it can be adjusted to assist offsetting the exodeviation for the benefit of maintaining single binocular vision. Since infants and young children seem to have a more pliable overall sensory-motor

innervating system than older children and adults, this could account for the fact the high AC/A ratio occurs most frequently among exophoric and intermittently exotropic youngsters. By this reasoning, the divergence excess exodeviation measurement results from an attempt to compensate for the excessive divergence innervation rather than from excessive divergence innervation as suggested in the preceding paragraphs.

EXOTROPIA

Exotropia is a constant divergent deviation that is usually associated with either a normal or low AC/A ratio. There is seldom a high AC/A ratio, except in the surgically overcorrected esotrope who had a high AC/A ratio prior to surgery, since there is no sensory reward to the constantly tropic patient for evolving a high AC/A. Unless the fixation continues to be alternated between the two eyes, the patient who becomes constantly exotropic prior to 10 years of age usually has amblyopia. In constant exotropia, suppression and ARC tend to be present, unless there is no binocular vision, as encountered in either the congenital exotrope, some congenital esotropes who become exotropic, or the patient who unfortunately has a unilateral abnormal eye.

MANAGEMENT

The divergent deviations are treated by several methods: compensating for the misalignment with prisms, urging the patient to compensate for the misalignment with fusional convergence, subtly stimulating the patient to compensate for the misalignment with accommodative convergence, or reducing the misalignment with surgery. The ophthalmologist's selection of treatment is dependent on the nature of the exodeviation and his experience with various treatment modalities.

EXOPHORIA

If exophoria is asymptomatic, it requires no treatment. Symptoms are rare in young children, and they tend to occur with increasing frequency in patients over 10 years of age.

Fusional convergence training by orthoptics is successful in most affected patients; this should receive top priority as the first method to alleviate the patient's recurrent symptoms. The objective is to enhance the fusional convergence amplitude by various techniques. Treatment is emphasized for distance if the exodeviation is greater at distance than at near; near exercise is emphasized if the exodeviation is greater at near than at distance. While doing the exercise, the accommodation should be controlled so that the fusional convergence rather than the accommodative convergence is stimulated. Small detailed distance targets are fixated for the distance exercises, and small print is read for the near exercise. Various combinations of loose 2Δ, 3Δ, 10Δ, and 20Δ prisms can be arranged horizontally to offer the following stepwise increments in stimulus to fusional convergence: 2Δ, 3Δ, 5Δ, 7Δ, 8Δ, 10Δ, 12Δ, 13Δ, 15Δ, 17Δ, 18Δ, 20Δ, 22Δ, 23Δ, 25Δ, 27Δ, 28Δ, 30Δ, 32Δ, 33Δ, and 35Δ. The loose prism fusional convergence technique used in combination with a Polaroid screen fitted over the television while the patient wears Polaroid spectacle analyzers ensures that the patient is fusing at distance rather than suppressing as the base-out prism increments are made. Bar reading provides an excellent method for ensuring against suppression at near as the increments of base-out prisms are made. Bar reading is accomplished by holding a narrow septum vertically midway between the eyes and the page; this obscures a different portion of the page for the right and left eye, but the entire page is seen undisturbed as long as the patient fuses. Various stereoscopic techniques are also available for stimulating fusional convergence. One technique involves using a series of stereocards in a Wheatstone stereoscope; increasing convergence is demanded as the patient progresses through the series. Another method is built around the Polaroid vectographic technique; a series of Polaroid vectographic plates (Orthofusor) are viewed through Polaroid analyzers. As one proceeds through the series of plates, progressively more convergence is required to obtain the stereopsis perception.

Whenever possible, accommodative convergence should be used to compensate for exophoria in the subpresbyopic patient by undercorrecting hypermetropia and overcorrecting myopia. Forcing 2 to 3 D of accommodation by appropriate spectacle power is usually well-tolerated in young patients; however, in older patients this therapy may provoke symptoms of asthenopia similar to those it seeks to alleviate, and the benefit is nil. Also, a medical method of stimulating accommodative convergence is available by instilling 2% homatropine eye drops; this increases the AC/A ratio, providing an increase in convergence to offset the exophoria. However, the symptoms of asthenopia and blurred vision that accompany this therapy regardless of the patient's age make this an impractical method for managing exophoria.

Base-in prism spectacles to compensate for the exophoria always have a place in the overall therapeutic regimen. These spectacles are particularly useful in both the presbyopic patients and the subpresbyopic patients, regardless of age, who are unable to increase their fusional convergence amplitude with orthoptic training. In this connection, there is an established clinical entity that is ideally treated by base-in prism spectacles. This entity occurs in young people and is lifelong; it causes symptoms during near vision manifest by blurred print and diplopia. Orthophoria or minimal exophoria is measured at distance, but a 12Δ to 18Δ exotropia is measured at near. Most significantly the amplitude, or range, of accommodation is conspicuously less than the norm for the chronologic age. Also, all fusional vergence amplitudes are obviously less than normal or almost nil, and, no matter how seriously the patient tries, they cannot be expanded. This near vision disorder presumably results from some deficiency in the optomotor reflexes. Accommodation, accommodative convergence, and fusional vergences are lacking, and there is no way to improve them. This patient should not receive prolonged orthoptic training. Presbyopic therapy with plus lens power is required for reading, along with base-in prisms to compensate for the near exotropia. The optic combination of these two therapies can be provided in reading spectacles; half-eye spectacles probably offer the best solution.

Surgery is seldom the answer for either distance or near exophoria, and it should be deferred until other methods of treatment have failed, unless the prism and alternate cover distance and near measurements are significant. Patients with either distance or near measurements that approach orthophoria are poor surgical candidates; an adult with approximately distant orthophoria and a symptomatic large angle of near exophoria is a particularly poor surgical risk. For such a patient with a low AC/A ratio, some ophthalmologists claim that resections of the medial recti improve the near exophoria without altering the preoperative distance orthophoria, but few have documented this claim of permanent improvement in near exophoria without this patient also having a disturbing postoperative distance esotropia. The exophoric patient with a large distance deviation and approximately near orthophoria, who never slips into intermittent exotropia while viewing at distance, is also almost never troubled with distance symptoms and rarely requires treatment of any kind, including surgery. The patient having a large angle of exophoria at both distance and at near (excess of 12Δ) and frequent symptoms does well with surgery, and it is justifiable to offer this treatment to him.

INTERMITTENT EXOTROPIA

Surgery is justified for intermittent exotropia if anisometropia or myopia has been adequately corrected with spectacles and if an eye still turns out intermittently. The best opportunity the patient has for complete cure is elimination of the exoangle prior to the development of suppression and ARC. If the patient is 10 years of age or older and suppression and ARC are not present while he is exotropic, then these sensorial adaptations to binocular vision will never develop, and the good prognosis for cure will continue unchanged. Until the patient attains approximately 10 years of age, there is always the risk that suppression and ARC will be learned while he is exotropic; once these are learned, they can always be retrained. These adaptations tend to be used and reused for any residual exodeviation, no matter how small, after surgery; eventually, the small exodeviation tends to build back toward the preoperative quantity. To prevent this discouraging result, the small residual postoperative exodeviation must be kept latent, as it is in patients without suppression and ARC. Attempts to prevent the suppression and ARC from ruining the immediate postoperative result by employing preoperative and postoperative orthoptics have usually failed. Therefore, the most logical therapy for intermittent exotropia is surgical straightening of the eyes as soon as possible after a successful evaluation of the alignment is made and daily recurrence of the exotropia is documented. This degree of urgency is not necessary in patients over 10 years of age, but to procrastinate in younger patients is to invite hardship in the future for both patient and surgeon.

Intermittent exotropia causes visual symptoms in patients of all ages, unless suppression and ARC have developed. Elimination of the exoangle by surgery is justified in the absence of suppression and ARC simply on the basis of removing the recurrent symptoms and disregarding the merit of preventing the onset of suppression and ARC. The divergent eye is cosmetically disfiguring and always a source of embarrassment to the patient. Regardless of the patient's age and state of sensorial adaptations to the intermittent exotropia, surgery is justified to eliminate the visual symptoms and bad appearance with which these patients present. The burden is on justifying allowing these patients to remain untreated and possibly deteriorate gradually from intermittent exotropia to constant exotropia, although not all ophthalmologists advocate this philosophy. Some ophthalmologists claim that since not all patients with intermittent exotropia manifest their exoangle as frequently when they are older as when they were younger, performing surgery on all young intermittent exotropes causes some patients to endure unnecessary surgery. This difference of opinion becomes an impossible argument because within the lifetime of one surgeon all of the facts necessary to support his position cannot be accumulated. For example, even if the child improves to the extent that the intermittent exotropia occurs less than daily, it may reappear twenty years later with more frequency. This could be the source of the disorder in the rare patient with a late onset who appears to develop intermittent exotropia in adulthood first. However, there is some merit in the argument for not operating on every child having intermittent exotropia since some spontaneously improve. Those with small exoangles are more inclined to improve spontaneously than those with large angles. Therefore, surgery should be deferred in the intermittent exotropic youngster whose maximal prism and alternate cover distance measurement is less than 15Δ, unless the exoangle increases or the intermittent exotropia increases in frequency and duration. However, for all patients, regardless of age, whose distance exoangle can be reliably measured as 15Δ or more, whose tropia recurs daily, and whose significant refractive error is compensated by spectacles, serious consideration should be given to proceeding with surgery. The surgery is usually recessions of the lateral recti or recession of the lateral rectus muscle coupled with resection of the medial rectus muscle of the same eye. As an initial procedure, the improvement provided by resecting the medial recti is usually not durable since the postoperative alignment gradually reverts to the preoperative status. Recession or resection of a single horizontal rectus muscle is a rather worthless procedure; it produces asymmetry of lateral gaze and little or no change in the primary position alignment. The choice of the initial surgical procedure used routinely by surgeons treating intermittent exotropia is rather evenly divided between recession of the lateral recti and unilateral recession-resection of the horizontal recti, with equally good results. Therefore, it probably is not important to argue the merits of either approach since the overriding factor that dictates the surgeon's choice is his confidence in the procedure. Recession of the lateral recti is advocated by some surgeons because it is neat and symmetric. Some surgeons believe that recession-resection produces a more permanent result than recession because the resec-

TABLE 13-1. Quantity of Surgery Suggested According to Exoangle

XT Angle	Recess LROU	Resect MROU
15Δ	4 mm	3 mm
20Δ	5 mm	4 mm
25Δ	6 mm	5 mm
30Δ	7 mm	6 mm

XT Angle	Recess LR and Resect MR

tion of the medial rectus muscle locks the eye in better alignment, preserving the benefit of the recessed lateral rectus muscle; they also claim that the asymmetric horizontal measurements produced by the recession-resection are minor and that they gradually improve.

Several factors determine the quantity of surgery used to correct the intermittent exotropia; however, there is still a base line quantity of surgery that is performed according to the distance prism and alternate cover measurements. The base line quantities are presented in Table 13-1. The table is read in one of two ways. First, by reading from top to bottom, it lists the quantity of surgery performed for exoangles ranging between 15Δ and 30Δ, showing the millimeters of recession performed per prism diopter of exoangle as the initial procedure; it also shows the quantity of resections of the medial recti that are performed per prism diopter of exoangle as the secondary procedure. Secondly, by reading the table horizontally rather than vertically and from bottom to top rather than from top to bottom, the millimeters of recession-resection of the horizontal recti of one eye per prism diopter of exoangle are apparent. For 40Δ, 50Δ, and 60Δ of exoangle, the surgeon selects an initial bilateral recession-resection procedure; he performs the same quantity of surgery listed for 20Δ, 25Δ, and 30Δ, respectively, on each eye.

Patients with a low AC/A ratio and also those having less exoangle in lateral gaze than in the primary position require adjustments in the quantity of surgery performed per prism diopter of exoangle listed in Table 13-1. The patient with a low AC/A ratio who manifests a near exoangle that exceeds the distance exoangle by 10Δ or more requires 1 mm more surgery per muscle than the table indicates. The patient having 10Δ or more reduction of exoangle on lateral gaze compared to the primary position requires 1 mm less surgery per muscle than the table indicates.

The surgeon who recesses the lateral recti should anticipate 20Δ ± esotropia in the primary position

on the second or third postoperative day (2). This is significantly reduced by the tenth postoperative day, and the immediate overcorrection usually disappears by the third postoperative week. The final result can be appraised by the sixth postoperative week. The surgeon who performs the recession-resection procedure must not anticipate more than a few prism diopters of immediate postoperative overcorrection. However, the surgeon who strives for straight eyes immediately after recession of the lateral recti consistently produces an undercorrection requiring secondary surgery for the residual exoangle. The surgeon who performs recession of the lateral recti must be prepared to accept transient postoperative esotropia for the first ten days to three weeks if he is doing an adequate quantity of surgery.

Undercorrections are more numerous than overcorrections according to the quantity of surgery advised per prism diopter of deviation (Table 13-1). Approximately 5 percent of those patients having recessions of the lateral recti according to Table 13-1 as the initial surgery remain permanently overcorrected compared to approximately 27 percent who are undercorrected and require secondary surgery. Undercorrections of 15Δ or more are reoperated with resections of the medial recti any time it is apparent that secondary surgery is needed six weeks or later following the initial surgery. If the initial surgery is a recession-resection, then the secondary surgery is a recession-resection procedure on the opposite eye.

Associated motility problems are treated surgically at the time of the exosurgery, except for overacting superior oblique muscles. A and V patterns are corrected by vertically offsetting the horizontal recti insertions, and overacting inferior oblique muscles are recessed. Overacting superior obliques are largely ignored in patients with intermittent exotropia because of prior bad experience in producing a postoperatively vertical deviation in primary position; this deviation causes a conspicuous torticollis in some patients.

Sustained overcorrection of the exoangle deserves prolonged observation, antiaccommodation therapy, compensation of the esoangle with prism spectacles, and occlusion therapy for amblyopia. This therapy is initiated by the sixth postoperative week, unless it is apparent that straight eyes occur when raising or lowering the chin because of an associated A or V pattern. Miotic therapy rather than spectacles is usually used for this disorder because within a few days it is apparent whether or not antiaccommodation treatment improves the esoangle. If the miotic does not control the esotropia, prism spectacles are prescribed that also fully correct the hypermetropia, incorporating base-out prism power equal to the esoangle. If there is a concomitant high AC/A ratio, a miotic is used in conjunction with the prism spectacles. The prism power is reduced as the esoangle reduces; the Fresnel prism is ideal for this because of the ease in making the change. The patient is reexamined at monthly intervals and if no improvement occurs within six months, surgical intervention is recommended. The surgeon is advised to follow the dictum of Cooper (3), approaching the case as though it were an unoperated estropia, unless a duction restriction is apparent in the field of action of the previously operated muscle which requires investigation and repair of this muscle.

EXOTROPIA

The management of exotropia includes treatment of amblyopia and surgery. Patients under 10 years of age may have their amblyopia improved prior to the surgery, but the majority of constantly exotropic patients either have alternate fixation or associated pathologic changes that explain the poor sight; therefore, only the minority require therapy for amblyopia.

Patients with congenital constant exotropia should receive surgery as early as 6 months of age, and sufficient surgery should be performed to straighten the eyes which usually are widely diverged. These patients are managed in the same manner as those with congenital esotropia.

Older patients with good vision in each eye receive surgery according to the same schema discussed for patients with intermittent extropia. Those with a poor seeing or blind eye invariably receive recession-resection on the bad eye. If the exoangle of the poor eye exceeds 30Δ, the surgeon will be unable to limit the quantity of surgery per muscle to the quantity that does not interfere postoperatively with the normal horizontal ductions of the eye.

The surgeon must do excessive recession-resection to straighten the large unilateral exotropia and

TABLE 13-2. Quantity of Surgery Advised According to Exoangle in Patient With Profound Amblyopia

XT Angle	Recess LR	Resect MR
40Δ	8 mm	6 mm
50Δ	9 mm	7 mm
60Δ	10 mm	8 mm
70Δ	10 mm	9 mm
80Δ	10 mm	10 mm
XT Angle	**Recess LR**	**Resect MR**

sacrifice normal postoperative abduction or be allowed by the patient to distribute the surgery between the two eyes; this means also operating on the good eye. The latter procedure is the best for the motility status, but it may be too disturbing to the patient. If the surgeon must confine the surgery to the bad eye, then the quantities listed in Table 13-2 are recommended.

In addition to the muscle surgery required to correct the long-standing large angle of monocular exotropia, the tightly contracted lateral conjunctiva and Tenon's capsule must be recessed, otherwise the muscle surgery is for naught.

An important factor that alters the base line quantity of surgery per prism diopter of exoangle is the size of the eyeball; microphthalmia requires relatively less surgery.

Youngsters having an exotropic poor seeing or blind eye that is cosmetically disfiguring should receive surgery by 4 years of age to prevent development of a psychologic problem due to the poor appearance.

REFERENCES

1. Burian HM, Spivey BE: The surgical management of exodeviations. Am J Ophthalmol 59:603, 1965
2. Raab EL, Parks MM: Recession of the lateral rectus: Early and late post-operative alignments. Arch Ophthalmol 82:203, 1969
3. Cooper EL: The surgical management of secondary exotropia. Trans Am Acad Ophthalmol Otolaryngol 65:595, 1961

14

Monofixation Syndrome

As the evaluation of strabismus therapy became increasingly critical, attention was focused on a relatively large group of patients who had a small residual deviation. This group attracted particular attention because, in addition to the consistent findings of a deviation measuring 8Δ or less and good fusional vergence amplitudes, there was a scotoma within the deviated eye that prevented diplopia.

Further interest was stimulated when it became apparent that some patients with small deviations had no history of strabismus. Anisometropia was identified early as a frequently associated factor in the nonstrabismic patients. Even more interesting was the discovery that some of the population free of strabismus and anisometropia had this same disorder. After it was noted that the common denominator in all patients with a small deviation was a small facultative central scotoma within the visual field of one eye, binocular perimetry studies on a control series of patients with straight eyes revealed that some of these patients also had a central scotoma. It was also recognized that the rare patient with a unilateral macular lesion, having straight eyes and peripheral fusion, has the organic counterpart to the unilateral functional facultative central scotoma just described.

Consequently, a group of patients, either with or without a small deviation, from varied sources constitute a specific ophthalmologic entity characterized by monofixation, due to the central scotoma precluding bifixation and active peripheral binocular vision. The entity is referred to as the monofixation syndrome.

Initial interest in the monofixation syndrome came by way of the small angle deviations. Patients with these small angle deviations were referred to as "flicker cases," by the British, because the cover test revealed a small "flick" as the deviated eye assumed fixation. This syndrome soon became confused with the normal fixation disparity described by Ogle (1) and others. In addition, this condition has been called fixational disparity and also referred to as subnormal binocular vision due to the lack of central fusion. In 1956 Jampolsky (2) described how some of these patients have greater alternate cover measurements than cover-uncover measurements, and he emphasized that this is diagnostic of the disorder. He described the suppression within the central retinal area in one eye of these patients, and he used this as an explanation for solving the diplopia caused by the minimal deviation. Jampolsky further reasoned that the peripheral portion of Panum's fusional space is sufficiently large to permit fusion with normal retinal correspondence (NRC). His opinion regarding the lack of success with orthoptic treatment for these patients to convert them to centrally fusing rather than suppressing the central rentinal area is clearly stated. Jampolsky et al (3) also noted the paucity of small angle exodeviations as compared to the frequent number of cases of convergent small angle deviations. In 1962 Jampolsky (4) referred to the monofixation syndrome as "fusion disparity." He implied that there is normal fusion, except for the absence of bifoveal fixation. He chose the term "fusion disparity" to separate a monofixation syndrome from fixation disparity which is a normal physiologic entity. There are two obvious dissimilarities between fixation disparity and the monofixation syndrome (Jampolsky's fusion disparity). The quantity of deviation does not exceed 6 to 10 minutes of arc in fixation disparity, but it may be as large as 8Δ in the monofixation syndrome. In fixation disparity, both macular areas function simultaneously; whereas, in the monofixation syndrome, one or the other macula does not function during binocular vision.

The impossibility of accurately naming this condition in accordance with the established semantic code in common usage for ocular motility and binocular vision was apparent early after the initial interest developed in this large group of patients. Appraised according to one respect, the patient was heterotropic, but in another respect, he was heterophoric. Any term selected to identify these patients was arbitrary. In 1961 the name "monofixational phoria" was applied to those patients with a deviation that was greater by alternate cover than by cover-uncover; it was claimed that the deviation was made partially latent by peripheral fusion while the image projected onto the deviated macular area was suppressed (5). At that time, interest was directed only to the small angle aspect of the deviations, and physicians were unaware that many patients without a deviation also had the identical sensory abnormality of suppression of one macula. Jampolsky's concept of NRC peripheral fusion acquired by the normal stretched out peripheral Panum's space was accepted, and the NRC seemed to be confirmed by the findings from binocular perimetry performed during dissociated conditions. The following significant facts about the monofixation syndrome were also added by this report were:

1. Anisometropia, in addition to strabismus, was established as a cause.
2. In some patients, neither strabismus nor anisometropia was present, and these patients were defined as having primary monofixational phoria; those with strabismus and anisometropia was defined as having secondary monofixational phoria.
3. Stereoacuity was first related to the nature of the fixation present: poor in monofixation and good in bifixation.
4. The facultative absolute scotoma was revealed by binocular perimetry.

In 1966 Lang criticized monofixational phoria as a name for small angle strabismus since there is a manifest tropia. Burian's definition of heterophoria is a "deviation of the eyes kept latent by fusion; heterotropia is a patent (manifest) deviation of the eyes in the absence of fusion" (6). Lang (7) proposed that the syndrome be known by the full name of microtropia unilateralis anomalo fusionalis, but he suggested that it be referred to ordinarily as microtropia or microstrabismus. In 1967 Helveston and von Noorden (8) used the term "microtropia" to describe an inferred small angle strabismus in their amblyopia patients with eccentric fixation whose amblyopic eye did not make a movement to assume fixation and who grossly appeared to have straight eyes. The majority of their patients were anisometropic. Since, by visuscopy, the fixation point was adjacent to the macular borders, they inferred that the strabismus angle was ultra small. Others can confirm these findings in many patients with the monofixation syndrome whose poor sighted eye either has not responded to amblyopia therapy or has never been treated; the syndrome occurs either as a

primary condition or secondary to strabismus, anisometropia (or the two combined), or a macular lesion. These patients seem to have monofixational orthophoria since there is no detectable shift in either eye by the cover test. Perhaps Helveston and von Noorden are correct in their assumption that in some cases there probably would be a discernible shift were it not for the slight eccentric fixation in the amblyopic eye; therefore, the patient is not orthophoric. However, use of the term "microtropia" is not justified to describe the patients without shift to cover-uncover when Lang previously used the term to describe patients having a deviation by cover-uncover. The group described by Helveston and von Noorden probably represents only one of many various groups of patients with the overall monofixation syndrome.

The semantic structure that evolved as a result of many attempts to label various categories of patients that constitute the monofixation syndrome has become a monstrosity. Surely such terms as retinal slip, fixation disparity, esophoria with fixation disparity, fixational disparity, flicker cases, subnormal binocular vision, convergent fixation disparity, pathologic fixation disparity, monofixation phoria, fusion disparity, strabismus spurius, microtropia unilateralis anomalo fusionalis, microtropia, and microstrabismus will vanish from ordinary usage.

There are three principal reasons for the past difficulties encountered in naming this syndrome: (1) an element of both phoria and tropia is present and whichever feature the author chooses to emphasize determines the selection; (2) fixation disparity, as a name for a specific physiologic process in binocular single vision, was plagiarized since the condition under discussion seemed to be a pathologic extension of the same process; and (3) the names selected revealed the lack of a total concept of the syndrome. As the syndrome was gradually put together, the lack of organization in naming each of the facets is now apparent.

Essentially, the patients with this syndrome have straight or almost straight eyes and a form of binocular vision in which their inability to bifixate is proven by a demonstrable scotoma in the visual field of the nonfixating eye during binocular vision. This essential monofixating feature and other associated features are always present, while others may be either present or absent. Fusional vergence amplitudes are always associated with the monofixation syndrome. The variable features associated with this syndrome are a history of strabismus, anisometropia, a unilateral macular lesion, amblyopia, eccentric fixation, orthophoria, phoria, small tropia, and possibly a larger deviation by alternate cover than by cover-uncover. The majority of the patients with the monofixation syndrome have gross stereopsis; occasionally, the only exception is a patient with congenital esotropia who is straight and has sensory and motor fusion. The name that fits all of these features is simply "the monofixation syndrome."

ETIOLOGY

Since patients with the monofixation syndrome have associated strabismus, anisometropia, a unilateral macular lesion, or an inherent inability to fuse similar images on each macula, it is helpful to consider each of these conditions as a separate etiologic factor. The monofixation syndrome is caused by any of the preceding four factors or by any combination of them.

Among patients with the monofixation syndrome caused by strabismus, there is a significantly greater frequency of corrected esotropia than of corrected exotropia. According to one author's experience (9), approximately 66 percent of the successfully treated horizontal strabismic patients are esotropes and 34 percent are exotropes; yet of the strabismic patients who develop the monofixation syndrome after treatment, approximately 90 percent are esotropes and 10 percent are exotropes. Obviously, the chances than an exotrope will develop the monofixation syndrome are much less than the chances that an esotrope will develop the syndrome.

The probable explanation for the greater frequency of the monofixation syndrome in patient with corrected esotropia than in those with corrected exotropia is the difference between the constancy and intermittency of the deviation prior to treatment. The patient with constant tropia looses the bifixation habit completely. The possibility of restoring it after deviation is eliminated appears to be directly related to the patient's age at the time bifixation is lost and to the duration of the constant deviation. Since esotropic patients prior to receiving therapy tend to have constant deviations with greater frequency than exotropic patients, one should anticipate that a greater percentage of esotropes than exotropes will remain monofixating patients after treatment. In a study made by the author at the time the deviation was brought under control, 70 percent of the esotropes and only 21 percent of the exotropes were constantly tropic.

It is tempting to conjecture that amblyopia is more prevalent in esotropes than in exotropes since in the study just mentioned, 40 percent of the esotropes were amblyopic and only 3 percent of the exotropes were amblyopic out of 100 consecutive patients having horizontal strabismus. Yet among patients with the monofixation syndrome, 78 percent of the esotropes and 57 percent of the exotropes are amblyopic. The latter fact suggests that the incidence of the monofixation syndrome as a final treatment status is increased in both esotropes and exotropes if amblyopia exists. However, it does not follow that amblyopia is the cause of the monofixation syndrome after the deviation has been eliminated. Evidence to the contrary was found in the fact that 24 percent of the patients with the monofixation syndrome were never amblyopic, and an additional 16 percent still had the monofixation syndrome after their amblyopia had permanently been cured by occlusion therapy. A more plausible concept is that both amblyopia and the monofixation syndrome result from the same cause, but the development of amblyopia requires one additional factor. Both are produced by prolonged and constant strabismic deviation in the infant or young child; but, in addition, development of amblyopia requires the constant exclusion of one eye from fixating rather than alternate fixation. Hence, not all patients with the monofixation syndrome following strabismus therapy have amblyopia.

Congenital esotropes appear to have a different reason for monofixating, despite the fact that peripheral fusion was acquired by early surgical elimination of the deviation. Congenital esotropes seem to have an inherent inability to bifixate. Some congenital esotropes obtain peripheral fusion if the eyes have been straightened by surgery at an early age, but they never obtain bifixation. Some congenitally esotropic patients who obtain peripheral fusion after their eyes have been straightened do not develop stereopsis. Although this result occurs in the minority, this combination of peripheral fusion and no stereopsis has been observed only in the surgically straightened congenital esotropes. Of the straightened strabismic patients studied, all others with fusion manifested stereopsis capability. It is tempting to speculate why bifixation never develops and why stereopsis occasionally does not develop in these patients even though the congenital esotropia is surgically corrected by 6 months of age. Perhaps there is some justification for Worth's suggestion that these children have a deficit in the fusion faculty. Proof that peripheral fusion is attained by early surgical intervention in a high percentage of congenital esotropes partially discredits this concept. However, there may be some merit in Worth's thesis since a defect in the faculty serving single binocular vision remains a distinct possibility. Regardless of how this observation is explained, none of the therapeutic regimens offered the infant with congenital esotropia to date has produced bifixation.

Anisometropia is another etiologic factor which presents an additional obstacle to macular fusion. A clear image on one macula and a blurred image on the other offers little reward for the effort involved in integrating the two into a unified perception. Presuming that similarly clear macular images are required during infancy for establishment of bifixation, one realizes that discovery of anisometropia at an older age is too late to expect bifixation to result from prescription of optic correction for equally clear images on each macula. Unless strabismus is also present, it is difficult to discover the anisometropia during infancy. The question that naturally follows is the age at which anisometropia must be optically treated to permit bifixation to develop. Too few facts are available to answer this question.

Occasionally, a child with 2 or 3 diopters of anisometropia and with minimal amblyopia demonstrates improvement in visual acuity of the bad eye simply by having glasses prescribed and no occlusion therapy. It can usually be proven that this child has bifixation despite the unequally focused images on each fovea. Therefore, the diagnosis of bifixation in this situation offers a prognosis for spontaneous visual improvement with spectacle therapy alone. This observation also suggests that minimal amblyopia and bifixation may coexist, which weakens the thesis that amblyopia is the cause of the monofixation syndrome.

A unilateral macular lesion is the organically defective visual counterpart to the unilateral functional macular scotoma that occurs in the binocular field of the patient with the monofixation syndrome. Many patients with only one functioning macula retain straight eyes; this apparently is accomplished by peripheral fusion. Binocular vision of patients with an organic scotoma is indistinguishable from the binocular vision of patients with a functional scotoma.

Patients with primary monofixation are a challenging group to study. One never ceases to be amazed at the large number of symptomless patients, unaware of the absence of bifixation, whose monofixation pattern remains unsuspected until disclosure by examination. These patients have poor stereoacuity, a monocular 3° facultative scotoma revealed by binocular perimetry in the visual field of one eye, and there may be a small shift in taking up fixation by the nonfixating eye upon covering the fixating eye. These patients are totally unaware of their disorder and without sophisticated testing techniques the examiner too would be unaware of its existence. The majority of the patients with primary monofixation have a small amount of ambly-

opia in the nonpreferred eye unless fixation is alternated.

Both patients with congenital esotropia and those with primary monofixation seem to have similar inherent defects that prevent central fusion. These latter patients seem to be unable to develop bifixation even though their eyes are straight and they have peripheral fusion; this is likewise true for the 6-month-old infant whose congenital esotropia has been surgically corrected. Since primary monofixation syndrome is frequently observed in parent, child, and siblings of congenitally esotropic patients one wonders whether or not the central fusion defect is predetermined in these patients, as suggested by Lang.

DIAGNOSTIC METHODS

The diagnosis of the monofixation syndrome is based on a scotoma within the binocular field and peripheral fusion with fusional vergence amplitude. There is usually at least 3,000 seconds of arc of stereoacuity (Fig 8-5) but some congenital esotropes who have the monofixation syndrome are devoid of stereopsis capability.

The cover-uncover test may be sufficient to make the diagnosis if there is a small fixation movement made in the nonfixating eye. The quantity of movement elicited by the cover-uncover test is recorded by simultaneously introducing the corrective prism before the deviated eye, which neutralizes the fixation movement, and an occluder before the fixating eye.

Regardless of whether or not the patient with the monofixation syndrome reveals a flick movement of the nonfixating eye with the cover-uncover test, a prism and alternate cover test is performed. All possible responses may be found in this group of patients: the patient may be orthophoric; there may be a phoria elicited only by alternate cover; the deviation may be identical by both alternate cover and cover-uncover; or the deviation may be greater by alternate cover than by cover-uncover (Fig 6-3). Therefore, no single response by cover test methods can be considered to identify this syndrome; however, there is never more than 8Δ of horizontal deviation manifested in these patients by cover-uncover.

The diagnosis of monofixation syndrome can be made only by sensory investigation. This investigation ideally includes a test to demonstrate fusion, a search for a scotoma, evaluation of retinal correspondence, and a quantitation of stereopsis.

Fusion may be tested in an illuminated room with the Worth 4 dot test at both 6 meters and 0.33

meter. The distance test projects approximately 1.25° on the retinal area, and the near test projects approximately 6°. Those patients unable to fuse the dots at 6 meters or 0.33 meter slowly approach them until they succeed (Fig 9-1).

The horizontal fusional vergence amplitude may be determined while the patient reads small Snellen letters at 6 meters projected on a 2.5° screen in a well-illuminated room. The base-in power and then the base-out power is increased, using a rotary prism, until the diplopia or blurred vision is reported. Both the break and the restoration points are measured (see chapter entitled Vergences).

There are several different methods for identifying the monocular scotoma in the binocular visual field.

WORTH 4 DOT TEST

One method is the Worth 4 dot test. A bifixating patient easily fuses the distant dots, but the scotoma in the monofixating patient obscures the dots projected into the nonfixating eye. Until the dots are projected onto a retinal area larger than the scotoma, the patient reports seeing either three green dots or two red dots. As he approaches the distant Worth dots, the retinal projection area of the images increases; and when it exceeds the size of the scotoma, suddenly the four dots are seen (Fig 9-2). The distance at which this occurs away from the dots allows an estimate of the size of the scotoma, since the projection angle of the dots is known for 6 meters. In patients capable of voluntarily fixating with either eye, the scotoma is illustrated in the visual field of either eye as they switch fixation from the green to the red dots and vice versa.

BINOCULAR PERIMETRY

Binocular perimetry is also used to study the scotoma. The binocular perimetric techniques may be built around a septum mirror or a projector apparatus that projects either color targets or Polaroid-treated targets on a screen that is viewed by the patient while wearing color filters or Polaroid analyzers. The projector technique is superior to the septum mirror technique because there is no target wand to distract the patient. In the author's system, a projector which shines a 1-mm sharply focused green light on a diffusely red illuminated screen is used. After placement of a red filter before one eye and a green filter before the other eye, the patient fixates a 5-mm black "O" target at 1 meter in the center of the screen. The screen has a 5° concentric black circle surrounding

the central target, and the patient is directed to centrally position the green target within the fixation target. The scotoma is manifest by the disappearance of the green test target as it approaches the fixation target. The position, shape, and size of the scotoma are determined by bringing the test target in along various isopters toward the fixation target and reporting when the test target disappears. Children move the mounted movable green projector as if it were a mounted gun. They find this binocular perimetric technique entertaining, and they quickly plot their own scotoma. Binocular scotometry is done in a room darkened except for illumination from the red light and green light projector. Since the red-green filters dissociate the eyes in a darkened room, binocular control of the alignment is lacking during this test. Hence, the scotoma is positioned in reference to the fixation target according to the deviation of the eyes disclosed by the alternate cover test. In orthophoric patients, the scotoma is centered around the fixation target; in patients with esodeviation, it is displaced heteronymously; and in patients with exodeviation, it is displaced homonymously. With this test, NRC is invariably demonstrated in patients with the monofixation syndrome.

Patients with bifixation have a dramatically different response to binocular perimetry than patients with monofixation. Those with bifixation superimpose the green test target on the fixation target without hesitation. However, unless the patient is orthophoric, the test target is displaced from the fixation target according to the point at which the visual axis of the nonfixating eye strikes the screen when superimposition of the targets is claimed. In contrast, patients with monofixation manifest frustration as the test target disappears during its approach toward the fixation target. These patients usually make many approach attempts before conceding that the test target consistently disappears at a point approximately 1.5° to 2.5° short of the fixation target.

The scotoma can be plotted by the green projector and red filter technique in almost all patients having the monofixation syndrome. The scotoma is probably always in the visual field of the nonfixating eye, but some patients find it impossible to hold fixation of the nonpreferred eye on the fixation target as the test target approaches it. As the target reaches the boundary of the scotoma, some patients surrender to the compulsion to switch fixation from the fixation target to the test target. Instead of the test target being within the scotoma, the fixation target is located there, and any opportunity to plot the scotoma in the nonpreferred eye is lost. Amblyopia is a definite factor that interferes in maintaining fixation of the fixation target with the non-preferred eye; the severity of the amblyopia is directly proportional to the degree of difficulty in maintaining fixation on the fixation target.

4△ BASE-OUT PRISM TEST

The 4△ base-out prism test described by Irvine (10) is another method frequently used to reveal the scotoma in patients with the monofixation syndrome. The patient who manifests a shift to cover-uncover usually gives a positive response for a scotoma with the 4△ base-out prism test, while a large percentage of the patients having no shift to cover-uncover respond negatively to this test. Possibly the explanation for this fact is that the mono-fixating patient with no shift to cover-uncover is more apt to switch fixation from one eye to the other when the 4△ base-out prism is placed before the fixating eye than to refixate this eye after fixation is broken by the sudden prismatic shift of the visual field. Patients without amblyopia and without a shift to cover-uncover are particularly prone to yielding a negative 4△ base-out finding. When the test works it is excellent, but there is always a large percentage of the monofixating patients who respond equivocally or negatively to this test.

BAGOLINI STRIATED GLASSES TEST

The Bagolini striated glasses test is another technique for disclosing the invariable scotoma in the visual field of the nonfixating eye in patients with the monofixation syndrome. The patient is taught to recognize his own scotoma and report on it while viewing a small hand-held muscle light 15 inches away in a normally illuminated room. The striations on the glass produce a sharp bright streak of light emanating from the light source across the entire visual fiield perpendicular to the glass striations. The glasses are positioned before each eye so that the streaks are perpendicular to one another in the binocular visual field. Oblique placement of the streaks is best, since this allows part of each streak to be on both the nasal and the temporal retina.

The glasses are positioned so that the streak seen by the right eye is at 135° and the streak seen by the left eye is at 45° (Fig 9-5). The transparency of the striated glasses offers two advantages over other testing techniques: first, the glasses allow a normal environmental test situation, and secondly, the examiner can evaluate simultaneously the ocular alignment and the patient's sensorial response. Most patients with the monofixation syn-

drome (if they are observant) see a scotoma as a gap around the light in the streak seen by the non-fixating eye (Fig 9-6). A little more of the streak on one side or the other of the light may be missing, and this is somewhat related to the deviation. Often more of the streak projected onto the nasal retina is missing in patients with esodeviation, and more of the streak projected onto the temporal retina is missing in those with exodeviation. The gap around the fixation light, projected onto a grid, indicates a scotoma of 3° to 5°. Until the patient's attention is directed to it, the break, or gap, is visually overlooked. It remains unrecognized in a manner similar to physiologic diplopia until the patient is made aware of it. In studying the scotoma in the visual field of one eye with the Bagolini striated glasses technique, the patient is encouraged to switch fixation to the other eye to observe whether or not the scotoma has been transferred to the visual field of the other eye.

A-O VECTOGRAPHIC PROJECT-O-CHART SLIDE

The A-O Vectographic Project-O-Chart Slide* (Fig 9-12) is another method for the study of a scotoma in patients with the monofixation syndrome. It is used in conjunction with a nondepolarizing aluminized screen. The polarized letters of the Polaroid Vectograph slide provide a rapid and dependable differentiation between patients with bifixation and those with monofixation. Each character on the slide has self-contained light polarizations; some are polarized at 90° to others. Viewed through analyzers, some images are made visible to one eye and invisible to the other, while some characters are visible to both eyes. This method provides a test environment closely approximating the normal binocular situation. The patient with bifixation reads the entire 20/50 (6/15)† visual line without hesitation, although two letters are seen only by the right eye, two others only by the left eye, and the remaining two letters by both eyes. The patient with monofixation deletes the two letters that are imaged only in the nonfixating eye. Occasionally, the monofixating patient who rapidly alternates fixation from one eye to the other reads all six letters, but he usually comments that as two letters disappear two others appear. This response misleads the examiner if the patient does not spontaneously comment about the ever-changing letters appearing and disappearing.

---

* American Optical Company.

† Metric equivalent in parentheses after Snellen notation.

CLINICAL CHARACTERISTICS

The majority of patients with the monofixation syndrome have amblyopia, but the percentage of patients with amblyopia varies according to the cause of the syndrome. In a study conducted by the author, 34 percent of the congenital esotropes, 67 percent of the acquired esotropes, 73 percent of the primary monofixating patients, 88 percent of the patients with combined strabismus and anisometropia, and 100 percent of the anisometropic patients without strabismus had amblyopia. Therefore, it is incorrect to state that the syndrome of monofixation and peripheral fusion is characteristically associated with amblyopia. It is more correct to say that the minority of the congenital esotropes, a majority of the primary monofixating patients, a majority of the patients with acquired strabismus, and almost all anisometropes with this syndrome have amblyopia.

Some monofixating patients view the world about them with trivial deviations of the monofixating eye, ranging from 1Δ to 8Δ of horizontal deviation and 2Δ to 3Δ of vertical deviation. Others manifest no detectable deviation of either eye by the cover-uncover test, indicating that during ordinary seeing the eyes are straight. Hence, the object of regard is simultaneously imaged on each fovea and, despite this, one image is ignored because the macula on which it projects does not function during binocular vision. Thirty-seven percent of the patients with the monofixation syndrome manifest no detectable deviation of either eye by the cover-uncover test. Therefore, it is assumed that only two thirds of the patients with the monofixation syndrome have a deviation that would allow the diagnosis to be made by the cover test. The percentage of deviation vs no deviation varies significantly according to the cause of the monofixation. Deviation occurred most frequently in those patients treated for strabismus and least frequently in those with anisometropia. The primary monofixating patients tested midway between these two groups.

Another clinical characteristic often found in patients manifesting a shift to cover-uncover is a greater deviation by prism and alternate cover (Fig 6-2) than by simultaneous prism and cover (Fig 6-3). Occasionally, the difference in quantity is striking, eg, 10Δ or more. Forty percent of the patients with the monofixation syndrome who have a shift to cover-uncover have an increase in the angle of misalignment when binocular vision is prevented during the alternate cover test. The probable reason for this phenomenon is the benefit derived by the patient who reduces the angle of deviation with his fusional vergence. The benefit derived by these patients, at least those having more than 8Δ of alternate cover deviation, is that the reduction of their horizontal deviation to within 8Δ permits continuation of peripheral NRC. The small deviation that remains does not provoke diplopia because only one macula is functioning at a time.

Monofixating patients are usually capable of easily overcoming their trivial deviations with their fusional vergences. Furthermore, some patients with this syndrome have no deviation even to alternate cover. Yet, even if there is no deviation or a trivial deviation up to 8Δ during binocular seeing, a macular scotoma is present in the nonfixating eye of these patients. At least in those patients whose nonfixating eye manifests no deviation to cover-uncover, the macular socotoma cannot be attributed to a suppression area that developed secondary to the diplopia. Even in patients who have a trivial deviation, it is difficult to accept the idea that the scotoma is a suppression adaptation to diplopia, since the fusional vergence amplitudes exceed the small deviation by a comfortable margin. In these patients having a deviation, it appears that the macular scotoma contributes to rather than results from the deviation. Supporting this concept is the fact that those patients having a larger prism and alternate cover deviation than cover-uncover deviation could have reduced the entire deviation so that nothing would have been evident by cover-uncover were it not for the location of the macular scotoma. If these patients were obtaining relief from diplopia by developing a macular scotoma secondary to their trivial deviation, they could have developed a suppression in the region of the retina that conformed to their larger angle of deviation elicited by alternate cover.

Suppression and ARC develop concomitantly in the strabismic child (Fig 8-6). Development of suppression is apparently a solution for the annoyance of diplopia in the central portion of the binocular field, but perpetuation of peripheral fusion with ARC is the solution for diplopia in the peripheral binocular field (see chapter entitled Sensorial Adaptations in Strabismus). However, patients with the monofixation syndrome seem to have neither suppression nor ARC. The macular scotoma probably is not suppression (active cortical inhibition) but merely an inability, or a forfeiture of a previous ability, to enjoy bimacular function Apparently, when this function is discontinued for a few months, it is not recoverable.

The evidence supporting the contention that monofixating patients have ARC is relatively difficult to assess. One problem is created by the strictness of the definitions which undoubtedly are tighter than the loose neurophysiologic process involved in retinal correspondence. According to the strict definitions of NRC and ARC, peripheral fusion is achieved in straight eyes with NRC and in deviated with ARC. Therefore, the retinal correspondence in the patient with the monofixation syndrome varies according to the presence or absence of the deviation by cover-uncover. In these patients with such trivial deviations, it is doubtful whether the neurophysiologic process required to change retinal correspondence from NRC to ARC really occurs. The definition of ARC may be too strict. Jampolsky (2) suggested that there may be a stretched out Panum's area which allows these patients continuance of fusion. This would make the neurophysiologic adaptation of ARC unnecessary. The physiology of NRC may be sufficiently elastic to allow peripheral fusion in patients having deviations up to 8Δ.

The range of the horizontal fusional vergence amplitudes for patients with monofixation is similar to that for patients with bifixation. In monofixating patients, there is no difference in the average fusional vergence amplitudes between those who fuse without deviation (NRC) and those who fuse with a deviation of 8Δ or less (questionable ARC). This finding is in contrast to the fusional vergence amplitudes, usually limited or nonexistent, found in strabismic patients having greater than 8Δ of deviation and unquestionable ARC. This fact lends further support to the possibility that the definition of ARC leads to incorrect reasoning about the retinal correspondence in the monofixation syndrome.

Patients with the monofixation syndrome who have stereopsis obtain this perception only from relatively large degrees of horizontal retinal image disparity compared to the excellent stereoacuity of patients with bifixation. Burian (6) states that stereopsis does not come about through horizontal disparity on the basis of an anomalous retinal relationship. The author's experience also corroborates Burian's experience that ARC patients whose heterotropia is larger than 8Δ do not perceive stereopsis. Yet, in the so-called ARC patients with 8Δ or less of deviation who can fuse the Worth 4 dots, who demonstrate a fusional vergence amplitude, and who simultaneously perceive the streaks on each retina created by Bagolini striated lenses, stereopsis is invariably demonstrated, except in a few congenital esotropes. This can be further evidence that, according to its definition, the diagnosis of ARC is semantically correct for patients having the monofixation syndrome with a small tropia by

cover-uncover, but that physiologically NRC peripheral fusion is present. Consideration should be given to redefining NRC and ARC, allowing for the possibility that NRC peripheral binocular vision may exist in patients whose deviation by simultaneous prism and cover tests is 8Δ or less.

Polaroid vectographs offer a convenient, accurate, and simple method for determining stereoacuity. The stereoacuity of the monofixating patient ranges between 60 and 3,000 seconds of arc. By contrast, one of the attributes of bifixation is superb stereoacuity; the bifixating patient has a stereoacuity range between 14 and 40 seconds of arc, with an average of 24 seconds of arc. Apparently, the basic issue in determining the stereoacuity is the scotoma in the visual field of the nonfixating eye. Bifixation allows the high resolving powers of each macula to detect minute degrees of retinal image disparities; hence, the stereoacuity is good. In monofixation, the retinal image disparity is detected by studying the images on retinal areas having low resolving power, which causes poor stereoacuity. Consequently, the same retinal areas with poor resolving powers are used to determine stereoacuity in monofixating patients with or without deviation. Derived from these facts, it has been stressed that stereoacuity is a reliable indicator of either monofixation or bifixation (11).

Much attention has been directed to the absolute scotoma in the nonfixating eye, since this scotoma is the single invariable sensory finding in the monofixation syndrome. The scotoma facultatively disappears within the nonfixating eye when its monocular visual field is plotted, unless an organic retinal disorder is the cause of the monofixation syndrome. The scotoma is absolute in that nothing is seen within the area as long as fixation is maintained in the opposite eye. Most scotomas vary from 3° to 5° in horizontal dimension and slightly less in the vertical meridian. Occasionally, the scotoma extends 1° or 2° farther onto the nasal retina in the monofixating patient with esodeviation and slightly more onto the temporal retina in the monofixating patient with exodeviation.

TREATMENT

The primary objective of treatment should be to induce the patient to become attentive simultaneously to the similar images on each macula, ie, to cease monofixating and begin bifixating. However, all attempts to accomplish this objective have failed. The treatment can be divided into managing motor and sensory problems.

Improvement of the motor problem is not usually necessary since the maximal deviation in the normal binocular seeing situation never appears to exceed 8Δ; this is usually within the range of being easily reduced to zero by the patient's fusional vergence. Occasionally, the alternate cover deviation in a patient may be a horizontal deviation of 20Δ or more; this causes intermittent diplopia when there is a lapse of the fusional vergence that was maintaining an 8Δ or less cover-uncover deviation. This rare patient may benefit from surgery designed to eliminate the alternate cover deviation. Prismatic correction of the motor imbalance may be used in lieu of surgery, but indications for this procedure are equally rare. Except for the rare patient who demands considerable fusion effort to control the large deviation, no benefit is derived from correction of the usually small alternate cover deviation by either surgery or prisms because monofixation persists. The motor imbalance apparently is not the cause of the syndrome.

Inasmuch as these patients have adequate fusional vergence amplitudes, there is rarely a need to prescribe fusional vergence exercises. However, if the exercises are prescribed, the amplitudes increase with the same ease as in the bifixating patients.

Sensory treatment includes monocular and binocular therapy. Monocular therapy is essentially treatment of amblyopia. Unless the monofixating child alternates fixation from one macula to the other, the nonpreferred eye becomes amblyopic. Occlusion therapy adequately manages this sensory complication. If amblyopia tends to return when occlusion therapy is terminated, partial occlusion is maintained until the patient is 9 years old. Occlusion therapy for one-half day is adequate to prevent recurrence of amblyopia. If glasses are worn, the lens before the preferred eye is occluded for half the day. Preferably, two pairs of glasses are provided; those with an occluder lens (Fig 11-4)* before the preferred eye are worn half the day, or after school, while those with the clear lenses are worn during the rest of the day.

Treatment of amblyopia, a monocular sensory defect, does not affect the scotoma which is a binocular sensory defect in the patient with the monofixation syndrome. The established orthoptic therapeutic approach for overcoming the scotoma due to suppression is training the patient to recognize diplopia, but experience has shown that the patients with monofixation syndrome are refractory

---
* American Optical Company Occluder Lens.

to learning to recognize diplopia, other than physiologic diplopia, or diplopia induced by displacing the image outside the scotoma with prisms. This is probably due to the fact that the scotoma is not caused by suppression (active cortical inhibition) but is the manifestation of the patient's capability to be attentive to only one macula at a time rather than simultaneously perceive the images on both maculas.

Anisometropic patients may be converted to alternating use of their monofixating maculas by spectacle or contact lens prescription. Supplying equally clear images simultaneously to each macula usually does not improve the chance for bifixation any more than compensating for the small deviation with prism spectacles, but some rare exceptions to this generalization have been documented.

PROGNOSIS

The most impressive prognostic feature of patients with the monofixation syndrome is their static alignment state. Over the years, their eyes continue to remain aligned as well as if they were bifixating, regardless of the associated factors of strabismus, anisometropia, a unilateral macular lesion, or absence of all three. Peripheral fusion alone seems to be just as effective as the combination of peripheral and central fusion in maintaining straight eyes.

Apparently, the monofixating patient has such a poor prognosis for ever becoming a bifixating patient that no therapy for the disorder appears justified, other than providing the ideal optic correction and occlusion therapy for amblyopia.

REFERENCES

1. Ogle KN: Fixation disparity. Am Orthopt J 4:35, 1954
2. Jampolsky A: Esotropia and convergent fixation disparity of small degree: Differential diagnosis and management. Am J Ophthalmol 41:825, 1956
3. Jampolsky A. Flom BC, Freid AN: Fixation disparity in relation to heterophoria. Am J Ophthalmol 43:97, 1957
4. Jampolsky A: In Haik GM (ed): Strabismus Symposium of the New Orleans Academy of Ophthalmology. St. Louis: Mosby, 1962, p 125
5. Parks MM, Eustis AT: Monofixational phoria. Am Orthopt J 11:38, 1961
6. Burian HM: Normal and anomalous correspondence. In Allen JH (ed): Strabismus Ophthalmic Symposium. St. Louis: Mosby, 1950, p 179
7. Lang, J: Evaluation in small angle strabismus or microtropia. In Strabismus Symposium. New York: Karger, 1968, pp 219–222

8. Helveston EM, von Noorden GK: Microtropia Arch Ophthalmol 78:272, 1967

9. Parks MM: The monofixation syndrome. In Symposium on Strabismus, Transactions, New Orleans Academy of Ophthalmology. St. Louis: Mosby, 1971, p 127

10. Irvine SR: Amblyopia exanopsia: Observations on retinal inhibition, scotoma, projections, light difference discrimination and visual acuity. Trans Am Ophthalmol Soc 46:527, 1948

11. Parks MM: Stereoacuity as an indicator of bifixation. In Strabismus Symposium. New York: Karger, 1968, pp 258–260

15

Concomitant Vertical Deviations

Concomitant vertical misalignment of a few diopters is not a rare occurrence. In most instances, good fusional vergences overcome the deviation, resulting in fusion. The best test to elicit small vertical phorias is the Maddox rod: the patient fixates a small, point source of light first at distance and then at near. The quantity of deviation is measured with the Maddox rod and prism, and the vertical vergence amplitude is determined. Treatment of the vertical error is justified according to the magnitude of the deviation and the symptoms it provokes. Vertical vergence amplitude training by orthoptics usually does not produce improvement. Compensating for a portion or all of the vertical deviation with prism correction in spectacles is often helpful in deviations below 10Δ.

Large primary concomitant vertical deviations not secondary to previous extraocular muscle surgery are rare. The primary concomitant vertical deviation must be differentiated from skew deviation, which is rather abrupt in onset, variable, and associated with symptoms caused by intracranial or labyrinthian disease. Orbital asymmetry associated with facial and cranial dysostosis is a common cause of concomitant hypertropia; the hypertropic eye is always on the side with the shallow orbit. Surgery on a vertical rectus muscle of each eye is the best treatment: one muscle has its vertical action in right gaze and the other in left gaze. Three- or 4-mm recessions of the appropriate vertical recti are adequate to overcome 15Δ to 25Δ of hypertropia; there is symmetric improvement

in dextroversion, levoversion, and the primary position.

Concomitant vertical and horizontal deviations are common. Therapy directed at both is ideal, eg, plus lenses for the accommodative esodeviation, which may be displaced in the spectacle frame to obtain vertical correction, or incorporation of vertical prism power with the spheric or spherocylindric power. Patients with relatively large deviations requiring operative intervention should have simultaneous surgical procedures on both the horizontal and vertical recti in the two eyes. Symmetric surgery is performed on the vertical and horizontal muscles to overcome the esotropia or exotropia combined with concomitant right or left hypertropia.

Concomitant vertical strabismus secondary to prior extraocular muscle surgery may be due to many causes. Correction requires determining the specific cause and surigcally eliminating it.

SKEW DEVIATION

Hypertropia that is not due to the usual causes and is associated with a central nervous system disorder or labyrinthitis should be suspected as skew deviation. The onset is abrupt, and the vertical deviation is usually large and variable. Skew deviation can simulate almost any type of vertical misalignment. It may be constant in all positions of gaze or there may be right hypertropia in one lateral gaze position and left hypertropia in the other. Skew deviation may resemble a palsy of a cyclovertical muscle so closely that an erroneous diagnosis can be prevented only by keeping the diagnosis of skew deviation in mind when there is an associated neurologic abnormality.

According to Cogan (1), skew deviation is most commonly associated with lesions of the cerebellum, brainstem, and labyrinth. The usual etiologic agents are cerebellar tumors and abscesses, acoustic neuromas, vascular lesions of the pons and cerebellum, and cerebellar herniations into the foramen magnum complicating platybasia. Skew deviation is rarely associated with demyelinating diseases.

Skew deviation is more common in unilateral lesions than in bilateral lesions; the eye ipsilateral to the brain lesion is usually the hypotropic eye. Skew deviation disappears once the etiologic factor is removed.

REFERENCE

1. Cogan D: Neurology of Extraocular Muscles, ed 2. Springfield: Thomas, 1956, p 133

16

A-V
Patterns

A-V patterns are manifest by a horizontal change of alignment of the eyes which occurs on midline upgaze and downgaze as the eyes are moved from the primary position. As the eyes move from upgaze into downgaze in A pattern, they splay relatively outward; whereas, in V pattern they splay relatively inward. The A or V patterns may be associated with orthophoria, esodeviation, or exodeviation in the primary position. Compensatory head postures that provide sufficiently improved alignment to permit normal retinal correspondence (NRC) single binocular vision are frequently found in patients having A and V patterns.

ETIOLOGY

Two principles have been advanced to explain the cause of the A and V patterns. According to one principle, contraction and relaxation of the horizontal rectus muscles occur as midline upgaze and downgaze is executed. There is some electromyographic evidence to support this claim. The other thesis attributes the A and V patterns to abnormalities in the cyclovertical muscles. Clinical evidence supports this explanation since overactions of the inferior oblique muscles are frequently associated with the V pattern and overactions of the superior oblique muscles are frequently associated with the A pattern. Furthermore, weakening the overacting oblique muscles more effectively improves the disorder than weakening the horizontal rectus muscles.

DIAGNOSIS

The A and V patterns are revealed by prism and alternate cover midline measurements, comparing 30° upgaze, primary position, and 30° downgaze. By performing the measurements at distance, the near reflex is removed as a factor in influencing the measurements. By raising and lowering the chin 30° the same distant target can be fixated throughout the measurements. The vestibular innervating system and tonic neck vergences apparently do not exert any influence on these measurements. Between upgaze and downgaze, a difference of 10 diopters in the horizontal alignment of the eyes has arbitrarily been declared sufficient variation to diagnose A or V pattern. Various gradations of severity exist, and there is not always an even gradient of change in horizontal alignment as gaze changes from 30° up to 30° down. In some patients, there may be only a minimal change between primary position and either upgaze or downgaze, with maximal change in the opposite gaze position away from the primary position.

Rarely, another variant of the A and V pattern is encountered; it is characterized by eyes diverging as they either elevate or depress from the primary position. Also, these patients usually have overactions of all four oblique muscles. The opposite condition of eyes converging as they either elevate or depress from the primary position has never been observed by the author.

MANAGEMENT

The only treatment for A or V patterns is surgery. Five surgical principles have been developed to explain how improvement is rendered.

WEAKENING OR STRENGTHENING HORIZONTAL RECTUS MUSCLES

Urist (1) suggests weakening or strengthening the horizontal rectus muscles, claiming the medial recti are most effective in midline downgaze since this is the usual position for convergence. He further claims that the lateral rectus muscles are most effective in midline upgaze since divergence is usually accomplished by looking upward from the downturned near seeing position to see something at distance. By appropriately recessing or resecting these muscles to alter their power, not only is the horizontal measurement in the primary position improved but also, theoretically, the A and V patterns is improved. For example, an esotropic (ET) V

135

pattern is improved with recessions of the medial rectus muscles, an esotropic A pattern with resections of the lateral rectus muscles, an exotropic (XT) V pattern with recessions of the lateral rectus muscles, and an exotropic A pattern with resections of the medial rectus muscles.

VERTICAL TRANSPOSITION OF HORIZONTAL RECTUS MUSCLES

Knapp (2) conceived the idea of vertical transposition of the insertions of the horizontal rectus muscles, proved its effectiveness, and popularized its usefulness in treating A and V patterns. He reasoned that vertical transposition of the insertions of the horizontal rectus muscles alters their scleral attachment relative to the rotation center of the globe, thus increasing the arc of contact of the transpositioned muscle in one vertical gaze position and decreasing it in the opposite vertical gaze position. Since the pull power of the muscle is related to the stretch put on it by the arc of contact, the horizontal pull power is enhanced and diminished in opposite vertical gaze positions, as compared to the unoperated horizontal rectus muscle. Hence, the horizontal rectus muscles become more effective abductors or adductors in the vertical gaze position opposite to the direction in which their insertions are moved. Stated differently, the transpositioned horizontal rectus muscles become less effective horizontal rotators in the same vertical gaze position as the direction in which they are moved. For example, the infraplaced medial rectus muscles are more effective adductors in upgaze than in downgaze or the supraplaced lateral rectus muscles are less effective abductors in upgaze than in downgaze. Therefore, an esotropic V pattern is improved with either recessions and infraplacement of the medial rectus muscles or recession-resection on one eye which also infraplaces the medial rectus muscle and supraplaces the lateral rectus muscle. The directions in which the horizontal rectus muscles are transpositioned for A or V patterns associated with horizontal tropia are summarized in Table 16-1. The concensus seems to be that the usual quantity of transposition is half the width of the tendon. Although some surgeons perform total-width transplants, they experience greater unpredictable results in horizontal alignment in the primary position. Half-width tendon transpositions yield 15Δ to 20Δ change in the A or V pattern between upgaze and downgaze. Full-width transpositions produce more improvement, but the unpredictability of the horizontal correction in the primary position plus frequent limitation of duction

TABLE 16-1. Directions in Which the Horizontal Rectus Muscles Are Transpositioned for ET and XT A and V Patterns

	Medial Rectus	Lateral Rectus
ET-V	↓	↑
ET-A	↑	↓
XT-V	↓	↑
XT-A	↑	↓

in the field of action of the transpositioned muscle limits the usefulness of this quantity of surgery.

Oblique muscle dysfunction associated with the A or V patterns is not changed by vertically offsetting the horizontal rectus muscles.

WEAKENING OR STRENGTHENING VERTICAL RECTUS MUSCLES

Weakening or strengthening the vertical rectus muscles was tried for correcting A and V patterns but did not pass the test of time. The principle that precipitates this technique is the secondary adduction effect produced by the vertical rectus muscles in the primary position. The total adduction produced by these muscles theoretically increases as the inferior rectus muscles contract in downgaze and as the superior rectus muscles contract in upgaze.

Recession or resection of appropriate vertical rectus muscles (3) reduces the A and V patterns. The changes produced are maximal in downgaze with surgery on the inferior rectus muscles and maximal in upgaze with surgery on the superior rectus muscles. The primary procedure recommended for the esotropic V or A pattern is recession of the appropriate vertical rectus muscles: the inferior recti for V pattern and the superior recti for A pattern are recessed. If secondary improvement in the esotropic V or A pattern measurements is desired, resections of the opposing unoperated vertical rectus muscles are performed. The exotropic V or A patterns require resections of the appropriate vertical rectus muscles: resection of the inferior recti for V pattern and the superior recti for A pattern. Secondary improvement in the exotropic V or A pattern is obtained by recession of the opposing unoperated vertical rectus muscle, as detailed in Table 16-2. Four-mm recessions and resections of the vertical rectus muscles are performed. The associated oblique muscle dysfunction is also improved by the surgery on the vertical rectus muscles. The horizontal deviation in

TABLE 16-2. Primary and Secondary Surgery to Improve Esotropic and Exotropic V or A Patterns

		Recession	Resection
ET	V	IROU	SROU*
	A	SROU	IROU*
XT	V	IROU*	SROU
	A	SROU*	IROU

* Secondary surgery. IROU, inferior rectus muscle of both eyes; SROU, superior rectus muscle of both eyes.

the primary position remains unaltered by the surgery on the vertical rectus muscles; therefore, surgery is also required on the horizontal rectus muscles at this time.

HORIZONTAL TRANSPOSITION OF VERTICAL RECTUS MUSCLES

Horizontal transposition of the vertical rectus muscles to correct the A and V patterns was first advocated by Miller (3). The adduction component of the vertical rectus muscles is enhanced or lessened, respectively, by transpositioning their insertions nasally or temporally, thus altering the effective moment of force of the contracting muscle relative to the rotation center of the globe. The change in horizontal alignment during downgaze is maximal with horizontal transposition of the inferior rectus muscles and the upgaze is maximally affected with surgery on the superior rectus muscles. For example, to decrease excessive convergence in downgaze, as encountered in ET-V, the insertions of the inferior rectus muscles are transpositioned temporally. The directions for the horizontal transposition of the vertical rectus muscles to improve the A and V patterns are listed in Table 16-3. The usual quantity of horizontal transposition is half the width of the tendon; this does not interfere with the vertical duction of the operated vertical rectus muscle. The horizontal deviation in the primary position remains relatively unaltered by the horizontal transposition of the vertical rectus muscles; therefore, surgery on the horizontal muscles is also required and may be done at this time. Although transposition of the vertical rectus muscles received an adequate trial by many surgeons, its general abandonment as a method of treating A and V patterns resulted from its relative ineffectiveness.

WEAKENING OR STRENGTHENING OBLIQUE MUSCLES

Weakening or strengthening oblique muscles is used by most surgeons to improve the A and V patterns. The rationale for this surgery stems from the secondary abducting action of these muscles; this action is classically considered to be present minimally in the primary position for both inferior and superior oblique muscles. The inferior oblique muscles become stronger abductors in upgaze than in downgaze and the superior oblique muscles become stronger abductors in downgaze than in upgaze. Consequently, V pattern is improved either by weakening the inferior oblique muscles or by strengthening the superior oblique tendons; the opposite is done for A pattern, as illustrated in Table 16-4. Since weakening procedures on the oblique muscles consistently improve the A and V patterns, they have great popularity. However, the weakening procedures are indicated only for overacting oblique muscles; this overacting may be lacking in A and V patterns. Weakening normal oblique muscles produces an underaction easily detectable in version testing; this is obviously an undesirable result.

Strengthening procedures on the oblique muscles are less dependable than weakening procedures and, consequently, are rarely performed. Resecting and advancing the insertions of the inferior oblique muscles nets little improvement in the A pattern

TABLE 16-3. Directions for the Horizontal Transposition of the Vertical Rectus Muscles to Improve A and V Patterns

	Nasally	Temporally
SROU	XT-V	ET-A
IROU	XT-A	ET-V

TABLE 16-4. Weakening and Strengthening Procedures on Oblique Muscles to Improve A and V Patterns

	Weakening	Strengthening
V	IOOU	SOOU
A	SOOU	IOOU

IOOU, inferior oblique muscle of both eyes; SOOU, superior oblique muscle of both eyes.

and insignificant reduction in the preoperative overacting superior oblique muscles. Tucking the superior oblique tendons temporal to the superior rectus muscles causes reduction in the preoperative overelevation of the eyes (resulting from overacting inferior oblique muscles), but this procedure often causes a postoperative vertical deviation and an obvious incyclodeviation in the primary position that was nonexistent preoperatively. Although the V pattern is improved by strengthening the superior oblique tendons, the same can be accomplished by weakening the inferior oblique muscles, with less hazard to the patient. Therefore, bilateral weakening procedures on the inferior oblique muscles are more popular than bilateral strengthening procedures on the superior oblique tendons.

Weakening the inferior obliques corrects 15Δ to 25Δ of the V pattern between primary position and upgaze, depending on the severity of the overaction of the muscles. The surgery does not alter the lower component of the V pattern between primary position and downgaze. Also, the horizontal alignment of the eyes in the primary position remains relatively unchanged (4); this is contradictory to the earlier principle that weakening the secondary abductors produces a relative convergence of 5Δ to 10Δ. Bilateral recession of overacting inferior oblique muscles is associated with a good prognosis, eliminating the overactions and not producing a cyclovertical imbalance in the primary position (5).

Weakening the superior oblique muscles is accomplished by tenotomy or tenectomy, including the tendon sheath, midway between the nasal border of the superior rectus muscle and the trochlea. This procedure eliminates 40Δ to 45Δ of A pattern; the top of the A (upgaze) is unchanged, producing an even increment of change in the horizontal alignment between the top and the bottom of the A (downgaze). The change in primary position is approximately 15Δ to 20Δ of convergence. This procedure should not be used unless there is a large A pattern with overaction of the superior oblique muscles. Even with the best surgical technique, a vertical deviation in the primary position is often produced postoperatively, and, in the patient who is able to fuse, a sustained head tilt may be adopted to compensate for the imbalance. Therefore, postoperative torticollis is a risk the surgeon imposes on the patient with fusional potential by performing bilateral tenotomies on the superior obliques. This risk does not prevail in patients without fusional potential.

Of the five methods described to surgically treat the A and V patterns, only two receive widespread acceptance: vertical transposition of the insertions

of the horizontal rectus muscles and weakening of the oblique muscles. Some consideration is given to the realization that recessions of the medial rectus muscles slightly improve the V pattern and aggravate the A pattern.

In patients with ET-A, the chin is often elevated, maintaining the eyes in downgaze (Fig 16-1). Pur-

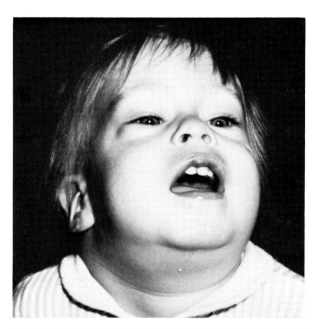

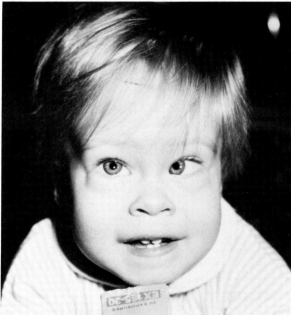

Fig 16-1. Compensatory chin elevation in patient with ET-A (upgaze and downgaze).

posely avoiding recessions of the medial rectus muscles and performing resections and infraplacement of the lateral rectus muscles failed in correcting both the esotropia and the A pattern. Recession of the medial rectus muscles, despite aggravating the A pattern, is necessary to improve the esotropia, and simultaneous supraplacement of the insertions prevents aggravation of the A pattern. This procedure has become the standard surgical approach for patients with ET-A of slight to moderate degree; this procedure corrects approximately 15Δ of A pattern. Large A patterns associated with esotropia are rare, and they are usually associated with underaction of the inferior oblique muscles and overaction of the superior oblique muscles. Tenotomy of the superior oblique tendons overcomes approximately 40Δ of A pattern but increases the esotropia in the primary position by at least 15Δ, requiring more surgery on the horizontal muscles.

In patients with ET-V, the chin is often depressed, maintaining the eyes in upgaze (Fig 16-2). Simply recessing the medial rectus muscles corrects approximately 10Δ of V pattern. Also, infraplacement of the insertions of the medial recti corrects an additional 15Δ of V pattern. Recession of associated overacting inferior oblique muscles corrects another 15Δ of V pattern between the primary position and upgaze. Therefore, presuming the ET-V has associated overacting inferior oblique muscles, recessions and infraplacements of the medial rectus muscles combined with recessions of the inferior oblique muscles corrects up to 45Δ of V pattern.

Patients with XT-A frequently have depressed chin compensatory head posture, and they keep the eyes elevated in fusing (Fig 16-3). They can receive 15Δ to 20Δ of A pattern correction with recessions of the lateral rectus muscles and infraplacement of their insertions. However, if greater A pattern correction is required and overaction of the superior oblique muscles is apparent, the surgeon may wish to tenotomize the tendons of these muscles. Since tenotomy of the superior oblique tendons corrects 40Δ of A pattern and reduces the exodeviation by 15Δ to 20Δ in the primary position, the quantity of exosurgery must be adjusted if the lateral rectus muscles and superior oblique tendons are operated on simultaneously. Furthermore, combining infraplacement of the lateral rectus muscles with tenotomy of the superior obliques would require that the patient preoperatively have 60Δ of A pattern, which is rather unusual. Therefore, the usual treatment of patients with XT-A is simply infraplacement of the recessed insertions of the

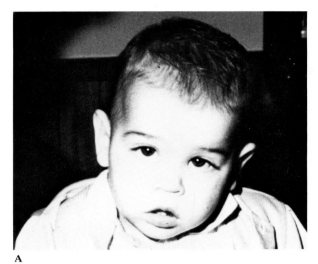

A

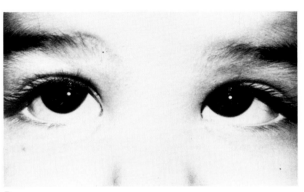

B

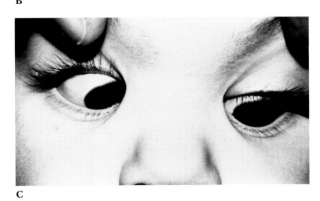

C

Fig 16-2. A. Compensatory chin depression in patient with ET-V. **B.** Upgaze. **C.** Downgaze.

lateral rectus muscles if the A pattern is less than 40Δ or tenotomizing the superior oblique tendons if the A pattern is 40Δ to 55Δ and if the superior oblique muscles are overacting. The surgeon should experience some uneasiness about tenotomizing the

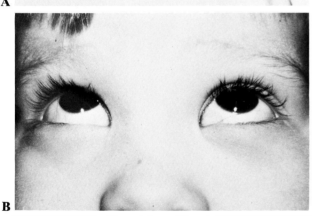

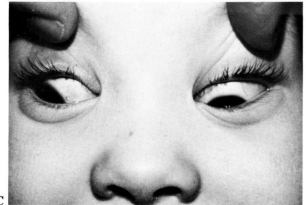

Fig 16-3. A. Compensatory chin depression in patient with XT-A. **B.** Upgaze. **C.** Downgaze.

superior oblique tendons in a patient with intermittent exotropia for fear the surgery will produce a postoperative imbalance in the primary position of the cyclovertical muscles with cyclovertical diplopia that is compensated for by tilting the head. The surgeon may prefer to disregard the large A pattern and the overacting superior oblique muscles in the intermittent exotrope, merely correct the primary position exoangle with combined recessions and infraplacements of the lateral rectus muscles, and accept whatever residual A pattern persists. If secondary surgery is required to correct the exoangle and if 15Δ or more of A pattern remains, the medial rectus muscles are resected and their insertions are supraplaced at this time. Tenotomy of the superior oblique tendons in patients with constant exotropia without binocular vision potential, having 40Δ or more of A pattern, and with overacting superior oblique muscles carries only minimal risk that postoperative torticollis will result.

Patients with XT-V frequently have chin elevation to permit fusion with downturned eyes (Fig 16-4). Surgery for XT-V correction is managed differently, depending on the presence or absence of associated overacting inferior oblique muscles and the quantity of the V pattern. If present, the associated overacting inferior oblique muscles are always recessed simultaneously with the lateral rectus muscles. This eliminates 15Δ to 25Δ of V pattern according to the severity of the overactions of the inferior oblique muscles, but the correction is only between primary position and upgaze. The inferior oblique muscles are never weakened if they are not overacting. Combining supraplacement with recessions of the lateral rectus muscles corrects 15Δ to 20Δ of V pattern. If it is necessary to correct more of the V pattern, the insertions of the medial rectus muscles can be infraplaced to provide an additional 15Δ to 20Δ of correction.

A and V patterns also occur in the absence of a horizontal deviation in primary position, causing a tropia in upgaze or downgaze. Oblique muscle overactions are usually associated with these types of A and V patterns. Overacting inferior oblique muscles are recessed in these patients, and the upper half of the V pattern is improved. However, tenotomies of superior oblique tendons in patients with overacting superior oblique muscles are associated with the high risk previously alluded to regarding the imbalance in the primary position of the cyclovertical muscles which causes torticollis postoperatively. The insertions of the horizontal rectus muscles may be vertically displaced without

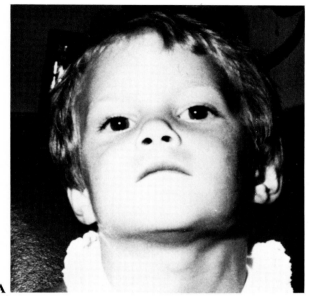

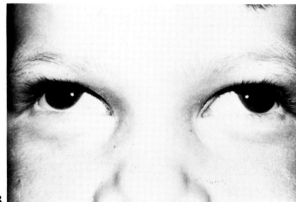

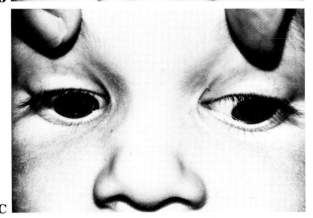

Fig 16-4. A. Compensatory chin elevation in patient with XT-V. **B.** Upgaze. **C.** Downgaze.

simultaneous recession or resection in order to improve the A or V pattern in these patients. Also, within this group of patients, one occasionally encounters the V pattern accommodative esotrope who is straight with plus spectacles at distance but esotropic at near due to a high accommodative convergence to accommodation (AC/A) ratio. Placing +2.50 lenses in a trial frame controls the near esotropia, but the near esotropia persists with bifocals because the patient must depress his eyes to use them. The V pattern causes the esotropia in downgaze, although the lower segment of the bifocal disengages the accommodation. In such a patient, the combination of the high AC/A ratio and the V pattern makes bifocals useless. Either a miotic must be used instead of the bifocals or the medial rectus muscles must be infraplaced to help this patient. The opposite of this disorder is the A pattern occurring in downgaze with straight eyes at distance and at near. Symptoms are caused by the exophoria that occurs when the eyes depress to do near work. These symptoms are relieved only by holding the near work up to eye level or by flexing the chin on the chest while doing the near work. The condition in this patient is improved by supraplacement of the insertions of the medial rectus muscles without a combined recession or resection.

REFERENCES

1. Urist MJ: Surgical treatment of esotropia with bilateral elevation in adduction. Arch Ophthalmol 47:220, 1952
2. Knapp P: Vertically incomitant horizontal strabismus, the so-called A and V Syndromes. Trans Am Ophthalmol Soc 57:666, 1959
3. Miller JE: Vertical recti transplantation in the A and V syndromes. Arch Ophthalmol 64:175, 1960
4. Stager D, Parks MM: Inferior oblique weakening procedures: Effect on primary position horizontal alignment. Arch Ophthalmol 90:15, 1973
5. Parks MM: A study of the weakening surgical procedure for eliminating overaction of the inferior obliques. Trans Am Ophthalmol Soc 69:163, 1971; Am J Ophthalmol 73:107, 1972

17

Oblique Muscle Dysfunctions

Oblique muscle dysfunctions occur in both the superior and inferior obliques. The dysfunction may produce hypocontraction or hypercontraction of the oblique muscles. Hypocontraction of the superior oblique muscle, often associated with hypercontraction of the ipsilateral inferior oblique muscle, is due to palsy of the fourth cranial nerve. Hypocontraction of the inferior oblique muscle is a rare disorder; hypocontraction of both oblique muscles is discussed in the chapter on isolated palsies of the cyclovertical muscles (see chapter entitled Cranial Nerve Palsies). Hypercontraction of the inferior and superior oblique muscles is discussed in the following pages.

OVERACTION OF THE INFERIOR OBLIQUE MUSCLES

Overaction of the inferior oblique muscle is manifest by overelevation of the adducted eye. It is a common enigma in the field of ocular motility. It may occur secondary to a weak contralateral superior rectus muscle or secondary to a weak ipsilateral superior oblique muscle. Most overactions of the inferior oblique muscles are unassociated with either the palsy of the contralateral superior rectus muscle or the palsy of the ipsilateral superior oblique muscle; hence, unexplainable overaction of the inferior oblique muscle not secondary to an attributable cause is termed primary overaction of the inferior oblique muscle.

The primary and secondary overactions of the inferior oblique muscles have different clinical presentations. Although the patient with primary overaction of the inferior oblique muscle presents with an overelevated adducted eye, there is little, if any, vertical deviation in the primary position (Fig. 17-1). The vertical deviation appears to be the only manifestation of the overacting muscle. An overacting cyclodeviation element is not clinically apparent. It probably would be more accurate to refer to primary overaction of the inferior oblique muscle as overelevation of the adducted eye.

In contrast, the overacting inferior oblique muscle secondary to a palsy of the superior rectus muscle in the opposite eye or of the superior oblique muscle (Fig. 19-6) in the same eye is associated with a significant vertical deviation in the primary position plus a manifest excyclodeviation. Although the cyclodeviation is present in the primary position, it is maximal in abduction.

The vertical deviation in the primary position in secondary overaction of the inferior oblique muscle usually ranges between 10Δ and 25Δ and the excyclodeviation from 5° to 10°. Consequently, the patient with secondary overaction of the inferior oblique muscle has sufficient imbalance in both cyclodeviation and vertical elements with the contralateral superior rectus muscle or the ipsilateral superior oblique muscle to produce a positive Bielschowsky head tilt test. In contrast, the isolated vertical element involvement in primary overaction of the inferior oblique muscle is associated with a vertical deviation in the primary position of between 0Δ and 5Δ and zero excyclodeviation. Furthermore, on tilting the head toward the right or the left shoulder neither the vertical alignment changes nor an excyclodeviation is produced.

PRIMARY OVERACTION

Primary overaction of the inferior oblique muscle apparently is not congenital. Rarely can the onset of this condition be recorded before 1 year of age. More commonly, onset is after 1 year of age; this condition may appear at any time during the first several years, most frequently appearing between 2 and 4 years of age.

Primary overaction of the inferior oblique muscle may be an isolated motility disorder or it may occur in conjunction with a horizontal deviation of the eyes. It seems to occur with equal frequency in patients with esotropia and in patients with exotropia. It appears with equal frequency in patients with congenital esotropia and in those with acquired esotropia. Furthermore, intermittency of the horizontal deviation does not seem to influence the frequency of this disorder. It occurs

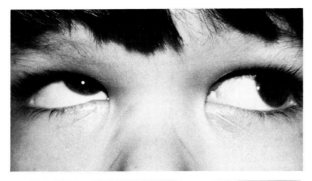

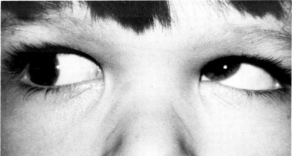

Fig 17-1. Primary overaction of both inferior oblique muscles.

with about equal frequency in patients with intermittent exotropia and in those with constant exotropia.

Primary overaction of the inferior oblique muscle may have its onset equally in the two eyes or it may occur only in one eye. After developing in one eye, it may gradually develop in the opposite eye. The dissimilarity in the degree of the overaction of the inferior oblique muscles may be temporary; with time, the degrees of overaction in the two muscles may gradually become equal. Unilateral overaction of the inferior oblique muscle occurs with sufficient frequency that the clinician is unable to make the statement that if one inferior oblique muscle overacts, eventually both will overact. Primary overactions of the inferior oblique muscles that are unassociated with any horizontal deviation of the eyes do not disturb the single binocular vision in the primary position. Depending on the degree of overaction, there is a measurable midline zone of varying size within which the eyes may make horizontal excursions and not disturb the binocular vision. However, the maximal horizontal excursion that is possible before the gradually increasing vertical phoria transforms to vertical tropia is recorded as the fusion breakpoint. At this point, diplopia is encountered. The patient usually responds by subconsciously limiting the horizontal

movement of the eyes to the extent that diplopia is avoided. Consequently, on viewing sideways, the patient is more apt to turn the head toward the position desired for seeing than to turn the eyes, except when he is startled by a visual or auditory stimulus located off to the side beyond the diplopic threshold.

Primary overactions of the inferior oblique muscles associated with a horizontal deviation are one of the mysteries of motility. It is often stated that the longer the duration of the horizontal deviation the greater the tendency for oblique muscle dysfunction. However, the congenitally esotropic infant who at a young age had excellent surgical correction of the horizontal deviation has the same chance of developing overaction of the inferior oblique muscles some years after the surgery as the congenitally esotropic patient who receives no surgery to correct the horizontal deviation until adulthood. Early corrective surgery for congenital esotropia does not diminsh the chance that the congenital esotrope will develop overacting inferior oblique muscles. According to one study (1), approximately 65 percent of the congenitally esotropic patients are destined to develop overacting inferior oblique muscles. Similarly, elimination of intermittent exotropia at a young age does not ensure against future development of primary overacting inferior oblique muscles. Correction of the accommodative esotropia soon after onset with spectacles does not lessen the chance for later development of primary overacting inferior oblique muscles. Therefore, one should question the statement that the longer the duration of the horizontal deviation the greater the chance of oblique muscle dysfunction.

Primary overaction of the inferior oblique muscles is frequently associated with a V pattern. In patients with congenital esotropia, the overacting inferior oblique muscles are usually associated with dissociated double hyperphoria or hypertropia. In some patients, the differentiation between overaction of the inferior oblique muscles and dissociated double hyperphoria is difficult. When the eyes have been horizontally deviated to the extent that the visual axis of the adducted eye is interrupted by the nose, the eye will deviate upward. This can simulate overaction of the inferior oblique muscle to the extent that in some patients it is impossible to make the differentiation.

The treatment of an overacting inferior oblique muscle is to weaken it surgically. Primary overaction of the inferior oblique muscle is not associated with an excyclodeviation, and weakening this primarily overacting muscle does not produce an incyclodeviation. Primary overaction of the inferior oblique muscle does not produce a significant vertical deviation in the primary position, and surgically weakening this primarily overacting muscle does not produce a vertical deviation in the primary position. Furthermore, unilateral primary overaction of the inferior oblique muscle is not associated with a positive Bielschowsky head tilt test, and this muscle does not produce a positive Bielschowsky head tilt test following the weakening procedure. In all of these respects, the primarily overacting inferior oblique muscle differs from the secondarily overacting inferior oblique muscle. The V pattern that may be associated with overacting inferior oblique muscles is improved by weakening these muscles, particularly between primary position and upgaze.

The inferior oblique muscles have a supposedly secondary abduction action when they contract to move the eyes from the primary position. For many years, allowances were made for a change in the horizontal alignment when the inferior oblique muscles were weakened. The esodeviation was claimed to be improved by 5Δ to 10Δ, and the exodeviation was worsened by 5Δ to 10Δ in patients in whom the primary overacting inferior oblique muscles were weakened. A study (2) has proved this claim to be erroneous. In effect, there is no significant change in the horizontal alignment of the eyes produced in the primary position by weakening procedures on primary overacting inferior oblique muscles.

In a prospective study (3), the various weakening procedures of the inferior oblique muscles have been investigated, and the conclusion is that the recession procedure is the superior method. The poorest method is a myectomy between the origin and the nasal border of the inferior rectus muscle. This is inadequate because of the significant recurrence of the overacting inferior oblique muscle which required secondary surgery in 33 percent of the patients. Three types of surgical weakening procedures were performed on the insertional portion of the inferior oblique muscle temporal to the inferior rectus muscle: recession, disinsertion allowing the muscle to seek its own insertional site, and myectomy between the temporal border of the inferior rectus and the muscle insertion. The tendency for recurrence of the overaction of the surgically weakened insertional end of the inferior oblique muscle was greatest with disinsertion while the result of myectomy was between those produced by disinsertion and recession. Repeat surgery disclosed that the disinserted or myectomized muscle had grown back to the original insertion site in most patients.

The worst complication occurring in patients whose overacting inferior oblique muscles were weakened was the adhesive syndrome. It was produced most frequently by myectomy at the insertional end of the muscle. Disinsertion produced a lower percentage of adhesive syndromes than myectomy. The adhesive syndrome was not produced by either the recession or the myectomy performed near the origin of the muscle.

The adhesive syndrome is manifest by a gradual development of hypotropia in the primary position in a patient who had no vertical deviation prior to surgery on the inferior oblique muscle. The hypotropia gradually increases over a period of several months to several years and may produce as much as 35Δ of vertical deviation. Furthermore, the patient is unable to elevate the hypotropic eye, and the traction test is positive for resistance to elevation of this eye. On surgical exploration of the hypotropic eye, the inferior oblique is not attached to the sclera. Instead, it is recoiled and attached to Tenon's capsule in the inferior temporal region which is thickened due to fibrofatty proliferation. This fibrofatty tissue extends over to the temporal side of the capsule of the inferior rectus muscle; this tissue is attached firmly to the muscle near its insertion. Presumably, cicatrization of the fibrofatty tissue, extending between the tissue of the inferior temporal fornix and the insertional temporal end of the inferior rectus muscle, gradually drags the involved eye further and further downward, causing the increasing hypotropia and diminishing active and passive elevation that are particularly obvious in abduction.

Surgical improvement of the adhesive syndrome is difficult; this disorder invariably requires secondary surgery on vertical rectus muscles following the liberation of the involved inferior oblique from its scarred Tenon's tissue and attachment of this muscle to the sclera. The adhesive syndrome is not produced by the recession procedure unless that portion of Tenon's capsule, which is the front surface for the intramuscular fat pad, is penetrated and the fat allowed to come forward and initiate the fibrofatty inflammatory response with adhesions extending from Tenon's capsule to the inferior sclera. The fact that this complication occurred in 2 percent of the disinsertions and in 13 percent of the insertional myectomies of the inferior oblique muscle and the fact that it may be many years between surgery and the onset of symptoms and findings should cause the surgeon some concern about the future if he chooses a procedure other than recession.

The surgeon performing the recession procedure should possess adequate skill and knowledge of technique and anatomy to make certain that the entire muscle is recessed and that Tenon's capsule containing the intramuscular fat pad is not opened. Adequate visualization of the entire insertion can be easily achieved with a sustained adducted and elevated positioning of the eye; this is easily accomplished with a 4-0 silk stay suture under the lateral rectus muscle attached to the drapes with hemostats. Exposure with a Desmarres lid retractor over the insertional site of the inferior oblique is possible through an incision in the inferior temporal fornix; this allows the surgeon to pluck the inferior oblique muscle out of its bed near its insertion by direct visualization rather than blindly sweeping a muscle hook under Tenon's capsule. The blind sweeping procedure has resulted in inadvertent myotomy and myectomy of both the lateral rectus and the inferior rectus muscles. Therefore, pickup of the inferior oblique muscle by direct visualization, visualization of the total insertion of the muscle, and 10-mm recession of the muscle produce significant improvement and do no harm to the patient's alignment in the primary position.

A 10-mm recession of the inferior oblique muscles may produce an overcorrection in slightly overacting inferior oblique muscles. Therefore, slight overaction of the inferior obliques should have relatively less millimeters of recession, ie, approximately 6 mm. Occasionally, primary overaction of the inferior oblique muscles recurs, even after 10 mm of recession. In this case, a further recession procedure is usually not helpful; myectomy of the inferior oblique muscle between the origin and the nasal border of the inferior rectus muscle also does not alter the trend of recurrence of the overaction. The only procedure to date that eliminates return of the overaction in this type of patient is total extirpation of the inferior oblique muscle (4). Thus far, total extirpation of the inferior oblique muscle has not produced any vertical deviation in the primary position. Even more surprising is the fact that the operated eye still elevates in adduction. Also, no incyclodeviation has remained more than a few weeks in the operated eye.

If the patient has unilateral primary overaction of the inferior oblique muscle, only this muscle is recessed. If the patient has marked overaction of the inferior oblique muscle on one side and only a slight overaction of the inferior oblique muscle on the other, both muscles are recessed. The markedly overacting inferior oblique muscle is recessed 10 mm, and the slightly overacting inferior oblique muscle is recessed 6 mm. An inferior oblique muscle which is not overacting preoperatively is never recessed. The principle that the surgeon should always weaken both inferior oblique muscles because sooner or later the unaffected mus-

cle will overact should be questioned. Undoubtedly, a large percentage of the patients having a unilateral overacting inferior oblique muscle that requires surgery present with the opposite inferior oblique muscle overacting soon after surgery on the first eye. However, those who do not have subsequent overaction of the inferior oblique muscle experience a significant underaction of the inferior oblique muscle that was not overacting preoperatively. Furthermore, bilateral weakening procedures on only a unilateral overacting inferior oblique muscle produce a vertical deviation in the primary position unless a change occurs soon after surgery that is equivalent to the development of an overaction in the muscle that was normal prior to surgery. However, not all normal inferior oblique muscles undergo this change, and in those that do not, the induced vertical deviation persists in the primary position.

Weakening procedures on the inferior oblique muscles are combined with surgery on the horizontal muscles if the misalignment is a combination of horizontal tropia and overaction of the inferior oblique muscles. There is no reason to perform separate procedures for the two different conditions.

SECONDARY OVERACTION

Secondary overacting inferior oblique muscles are the result of secondary changes, ie, hypertrophy or contracture. Hypertrophy occurs in the inferior oblique muscle when its yoke (contralateral superior rectus muscle) is palsied and the palsied eye is preferred for fixation. For example, in the patient with palsy of the right superior rectus muscle and a dominant right eye, the left inferior oblique muscle receives excessive innervation. The chronic hypertonus caused by excessive innervation produces hypertrophy of this muscle.

Contracture results in the inferior oblique muscle when it is the direct antagonist of the paretic ipsilateral superior oblique muscle and the uninvolved eye is preferred for fixation. For example, in the patient with palsy of the left superior oblique muscle and a dominant right eye, the tone of the left inferior oblique muscle in the primary position is not offset by the weak antagonistic tone of the left superior oblique muscle. Consequently, the globe persistently remains elevated and the left inferior oblique muscle is chronically more contracted than the left superior oblique muscle; this causes the left inferior oblique muscle to become shortened.

Regardless of whether or not there is hypertrophy or contracture of the secondary overacting inferior oblique muscle, a significant vertical deviation develops in the primary position that increases in the field of vertical action of the inferior oblique muscle. There is also an excyclodeviation in the primary position. A V pattern is usually associated with the secondary overacting inferior oblique muscle.

The secondary overacting inferior oblique muscle requires time to develop after the onset of the palsied superior rectus muscle or the superior oblique muscle. Usually the time required to produce this change is in excess of six months, although there are exceptions to this; some patients show the earliest signs of hypertrophy or contracture of the inferior oblique muscle within several weeks after the onset of the palsy.

The treatment of secondary overaction of the inferior oblique muscle is to weaken it, and the ideal procedure is recession. This should be performed prior to tucking the palsied superior oblique tendon or resecting the palsied superior rectus muscle. Also, recession of the hypertrophied or contractured inferior oblique muscle should be performed prior to weakening the yoke muscle.

OVERACTION OF THE SUPERIOR OBLIQUE MUSCLES

Overaction of the superior oblique muscles is not comparably divided into primary and secondary, as with the overacting inferior oblique muscles. Palsies of the inferior rectus or inferior oblique muscles are so rare that it is difficult to substantiate a difference between the clinical presentations of overacting superior oblique muscles resulting from this source and the primary overacting inferior oblique muscle. Therefore, this discussion pertains only to the primary type of overacting superior oblique muscles (Fig 17-2). Unilateral overaction of the superior oblique muscle produces a vertical deviation in the primary position. Bilateral overacting superior oblique muscles usually have little vertical deviation in the primary position, unless the overaction is maximal in one eye and minimal in the other. The patient has a hypotropia in the primary position of the eye with the maximal overacting superior oblique muscle. Neither incyclodeviation is produced nor is the Bielschowsky head tilt test rendered positive in patients having overacting superior oblique muscles. Overacting superior oblique muscles produce a significant A pattern and also produce an exoalignment of the eyes in the primary position.

Overacting superior oblique muscles apparently are acquired since they are not seen in infants. They are usually associated with a horizontal deviation, more frequently with exodeviation than

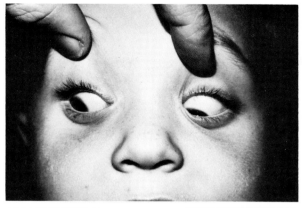

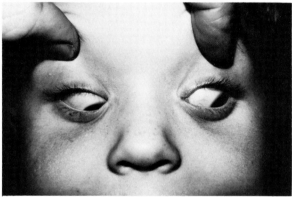

Fig 17-2. Primary overaction of both superior oblique muscles.

with esodeviation. Occasionally, overacting superior oblique muscles are found in patients free of any horizontal deviation in the primary position.

The treatment of overacting superior obliques is tenotomy of the superior oblique tendon nasal to the superior rectus muscle, making no attempt to spare transection of the sheath. Despite incising the tendon and sheath, the superior oblique muscle continues to function. The adducted eye still normally depresses. Weakening both superior oblique tendons changes the horizontal alignment in the primary position by approximately 15Δ to 20Δ, reducing the exodeviation or increasing the esodeviation. Also, it significantly improves the A pattern as much as 40Δ to 45Δ.

Often, a vertical deviation is produced in the primary position which did not exist preoperatively. This causes vertical diplopia in patients having single binocular vision; this can be eliminated by tilting the head to one shoulder or the other. This disappointing vertical deviation with torticollis is difficult to repair. Therefore, there is some danger in performing superior oblique tenotomies in patients with fusion.

For horizontal tropias associated with overacting superior oblique muscles, the superior obliques are operated on at the same time as the horizontal muscles.

REFERENCES

1. Manson R, Parks MM: Associated findings in congenital esotropia, to be published

2. Stager D, Parks MM: Inferior oblique weakening procedures: Effect on primary position horizontal alignment. Am J Ophthalmol 90:15, 1973

3. Parks MM: A study of the weakening surgical procedure for eliminating overaction of the inferior obliques. Trans Am Ophthalmol Soc 69:163, 1971

4. Parks MM: Total extirpation of the recurrent overacting inferior oblique muscle after maximal recession, to be published

18

Dissociated Hyperdeviations

A dissociated hyperdeviation is the upward turning of the nonfixating eye. It may be unilateral or bilateral; if it is bilateral, it is referred to as dissociated double hyperdeviation. If it is unilateral, it is identified by the nonfixating eye that elevates: either right dissociated hyperdeviation or left dissociated hyperdeviation. Dissociated double hyperdeviation is synonymous with alternating sursumduction which describes the upturning movement of each eye as the cover-uncover test is performed.

A separate chapter on the dissociated hyperdeviations is necessarily brief, but this is no reflection on its frequency or importance. Dissociated hyperdeviation is a frequently encountered motility disorder which causes considerable confusion to all except the most experienced clinicians. It can be confused with many other disorders of the vertical muscles, and until its nature is totally understood and appreciated, errors in diagnosis of and therapy for imbalances in the vertical muscles are easily committed.

Dissociated double hyperdeviation is almost always a bilateral condition; however, on rare occasions, a unilateral disorder may be encountered. The frequency of the diagnosis of unilateral versus bilateral involvement is somewhat related to the thoroughness of the examination and to how strictly the clinical findings are interpreted as they relate to the descriptive term of dissociated hyperdeviation. The term is inappropriate when it is applied to the majority of the cases because there is a cyclodeviation in addition to the hyperdeviation. It would probably be more appropriate to term this condition "dissociated cyclohyperdeviation," but because of the deeply established vertical designation for this entity, the author is not proposing that this name change be made. However, there is more to the deviation than simply a vertical movement.

Dissociated hyperdeviations may present either as a phoria or a tropia, depending on the presence or absence of single binocular vision. It always presents in the form of monofixation. For the past several years, all documented cases tested have never revealed bifixation. Therefore, if the patient has dissociated hyperphoria, it is dissociated monofixating hyperphoria. Like all patients with the monofixation syndrome, those with dissociated monofixating hyperphoria may have either a small manifest vertical deviation in the primary position or none that can be appreciated by the cover-uncover test. If there is a deviation while maintaining normal retinal correspondence single binocular vision, the vertical deviation is usually less than 5Δ.

Dissociated hyperphoria is recognized by the upward deviation of the covered eye. If this is dissociated double hyperphoria, either eye moves upward when covered. On alternate cover, either eye turns upward when covered, and the uncovered eye moves downward to fixate as the cover is shifted from side to side. To perform the cover test properly while investigating dissociated hyperdeviation, the cover should be remote from the patient's eyes. By breaking fixation with the cover approximately 25 cm in front of the patient, the examiner can obliquely visualize the patient's eyes behind the cover and observe the upward and downward movement as the cover is placed and removed from in front of either eye. An examiner should also provide good illumination of the patient's eyes and magnification if necessary to observe the crypts of the iris which are most revealing of the cyclodeviation that occurs simultaneously with the hyperdeviation. When the eye is covered it extorts, and as the eye is uncovered, it intorts. A seesaw vertical effect is observed during an alternate cover test; the covered eye moves up and the uncovered eye moves down to fixate. Dextrocycloversion and levocycloversion occur simultaneously with the positive and negative vertical vergences during the alternate cover test. Consequently, this disorder produces simultaneous opposite vertical movements and identical cyclomovements of the two eyes. These complex movements can be seen advantageously with the remote cover test just described. Variations in the vertical deviations and the cyclodeviations are encountered in different patients. The vertical deviations may be the major conspicuous component of the clinical picture in one patient, whereas, the cyclodeviations may be the major clinical finding in another patient. The deviations may be symmetrical in quantity in the right and the left eye or they may be negligible in one eye and maximal in the other. Occasionally, there may be total absence of the cyclodeviation or at least an apparent absence; this should be questioned because microscopic or electronic testing may prove its presence. Similarly, the cyclodeviation or the vertical deviation may appear to be present only in one eye. However, this must be questioned because perhaps more sophisticated testing would prove that the condition is bilateral but so minimal in one eye that it is impossible to detect it by gross visual observation. Also, the vertical deviation may be present in both eyes and a cyclodeviation apparent only in one eye or vice versa. The vertical deviation is seldom the same in the two eyes. As the alternate cover test is repeated, it becomes almost impossible to record in prism diopters the quantity of vertical deviation that occurs because of the variability as the test is continued. Therefore, it is practically impossible to obtain repeatable quantitative measurements of the vertical deviation in these patients.

According to the established semantic system, dissociated hypertropia differs from dissociated hyperphoria in that the cover test discloses a deviation. Semantically, this strict separation of patients with small dissociated hyperdeviation probably creates more problems than it solves, since many of these patients have a small manifest deviation of 4Δ or less. However, most of these patients reveal a greater hyperdeviation in the nonfixating eye when it is covered than when it is uncovered. This indicates that a certain component of the hyperdeviation is manifest up to approximately 4Δ within the framework of peripheral fusion, and the full deviation is revealed when peripheral fusion is interrupted by the cover test. Manifest hyperdeviations in excess of 5Δ usually represent the total deviation; placing the cover before the hypertrophic eye reveals no additional hyperdeviation. In patients with dissociated double hypertropia and severe amblyopia, the amblyopic eye which persistently manifests the hypertropia may remain high after the cover has been placed before the fixating eye.

An interesting finding known as the Bielschowsky phenomenon is frequently encountered in the dissociated hyperdeviation. This phenomenon is manifest as a downward movement of the high eye, which may infraduct to a point lower than the fixating eye, after the illumination entering the fixating eye has been sufficiently altered as compared with the quantity of illumination entering

the nonfixating eye. This can be accomplished by either reducing or increasing the illumination entering the fixating eye without disturbing the base illumination entering the nonfixating eye. One employs a photometric wedge, a series of filters having varied density arranged in a gradient manner on a filter rack, or polarized analyzers rotating in opposite directions until sufficient illumination entering the fixating eye is reduced to trigger the phenomenon. When the stimulus threshold is attained in the fixating eye, the examiner notes that the patient's nonfixating eye is making the downward movement. The same phenomenon can be produced by increasing the illumination only to the fixating eye; when the illumination exceeds the stimulus threshold, the phenomenon is triggered. This test is performed easily on patients with dissociated hypertropia, but it is slightly more difficult in those with dissociated hyperphoria. The patient with hyperphoria must have the hyperdeviation manifest by covering an eye, and the covered eye must be observed for the Bielschowsky phenomenon as the illumination entering the fixating eye is altered.

A phenomenon similar to the Bielschowsky phenomenon occurs in latent nystagmus. Latent nystagmus is converted to manifest nystagmus by raising or lowering the illumination presented to one eye. Also, dissociated hyperdeviation occurs frequently in association with latent nystagmus. Because of these similarities, both latent nystagmus and dissociated hyperdeviations have been attributed to some peculiar abnormal manifestation of the atavistic light reflex (1).

Dissociated hyperdeviation is most frequently encountered in patients with congenital esotropia; however, it can be encountered in those with orthophoria, exodeviation, and intermittent esodeviation. Dissociated hyperdeviation has not been observed by the author in the congenital esotrope until 8 months of age. The patient is usually not sufficiently cooperative until after 2 years of age for the refined examination required to detect dissociated hyperdeviation. Also, because most congenital esotropes have rather large angles of esotropia, the gross horizontal movements produced by the alternate cover test are such that a small hyperdeviation and cyclodeviation are not detectable. The eyes are positioned horizontally so that a small dissociated hyperdeviation can be easily detected only after the large angle of esotropia is surgically eliminated. Dissociated hyperdeviation probably is not present in 100 percent of the congenital esotropes, but it has been documented (2) in at least 70 percent of them; this is probably too conservative because not all patients had an extremely careful observation made specifically to determine the presence of dissociated hyperdeviation. Only those patients with conspicuous hyperdeviation were recorded as having this associated finding. A more thorough study with magnification and good illumination would have probably disclosed that 85 to 90 percent had dissociated hyperdeviation. The most impressive fact concerning congenital esotropia and dissociated hyperdeviation is the almost complete association between these two disorders. Because of this association, it is suggestive that dissociated hyperdeviations are genetically determined since, as stated in the chapter entitled Esodeviations, the frequency of congenital esotropia in multiple family members is high.

Eventually, congenital esotropes frequently develop overacting inferior oblique muscles; this complication of congenital esotropia is usually not evident until 1 year of age or older. Early surgery neither reduces the chance that overacting inferior oblique muscles nor dissociated double hyperdeviation will occur. Clinically, the association of both dissociated hyperdeviation and overacting inferior oblique muscles presents a diagnostic complication. The overelevation of the adducting eye, which is identified as a result of an overacting inferior oblique muscle, may be confused with dissociated hyperdeviation that converts hyperphoria to hypertropia when the nose, acting as a cover in the cover-uncover test, interferes with the fixation of the adducting eye (Fig 18-1). In some patients, it is impossible to determine whether the upturning adducted eye is due to an overacting inferior oblique muscle or dissociated hyperdeviation.

Unless the cosmetic aspect of the dissociated hypertropia is disturbing, one need not consider treatment; however, disfigurement is fairly common. The patient manifesting dissociated hypertropia suffers no symptoms because there is no binocular vision during the tropic manifestation. Some patients have intermittent dissociated hypertropia and maintain peripheral binocular vision while the deviation remains latent, and they experience no binocular vision when the dissociated hyperdeviation is manifest. Young children with intermittent dissociated hyperdeviation maintain phoria when they are well and rested, but they lapse into the manifest hypertropia with its cosmetic disfigurement when they are fatigued, ill, or emotionally disturbed. If the manifest hypertropia is much less in duration than the latent hyperphoria, nothing should be done therapeutically in the hope that eventually the hypertropic phase will diminish and even disappear; this frequently occurs by the time the patient reaches 8 years of age. If the patient also has overacting inferior oblique muscles, recessing the overacting inferior oblique muscles does not alter the cosmetic defect created by the manifest hyperdeviation in the primary position. If the deviation and cosmetic effect of the hyperdeviation in the primary position are significant enough to justify surgery, the best surgical correction is resection of the inferior rectus muscle of the involved eye. If the patient has good vision in

Fig 18-1. A and **B.** Dissociated double hyperdeviation manifest by cover-uncover in the primary position. **C** and **D.** Overacting inferior oblique muscles manifest by overelevation of the adducting eye.

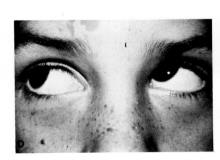
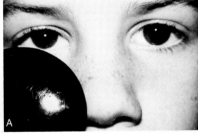
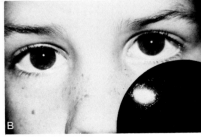
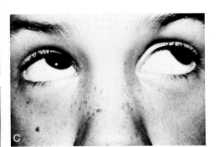

each eye and frequently alternates the fixation, the inferior rectus muscle should be resected in each eye. The benefit offered by resection of the inferior rectus muscle is probably one of simply anchoring the eye in a downturned position which is provided by tightening the inferior rectus muscle. Weakening the elevating muscles, the superior rectus muscle and the inferior oblique muscle, offers little if any improvement in the manifest dissociated hyperdeviation as compared with the resection of the inferior rectus muscle. The inferior rectus muscle should be resected at least 4 mm; if the deviation is moderate, 6 mm, and if large, 8 mm of the inferior rectus muscle must be resected. Resecting only one inferior rectus muscle usually transfers the overt hypertropia to the other eye; this discouraging result can be prevented with bilateral surgery.

REFERENCES

1. Cogan D: Neurology of Extraocular Muscles, ed 2. Springfield: Thomas, 1956, p 133
2. Manson R, Parks MM: Associated findings in congenital esotropia, to be published

19

Cranial Nerve Palsies

A palsy of any one of the three motor nerves that supply the extraocular muscles presents with characteristic findings affecting the ocular motility. A single nerve may be involved or there may be a degree of bilateral involvement in either the third, fourth, or sixth nerves or various combinations of them may be involved in the lesion. The palsy may be congenital due to some defect in the development of the nucleus or motor nerve fibers or it may be acquired. The lesion is located in or beyond the nucleus. If the motor fibers are affected, they may be interrupted either intramedullarly or extramedullarly; if extramedullarly, the involvement may be intracranial (within the foramen through which the nerve exits from the cranium) or extracranial (intraorbital).

THIRD NERVE PALSY

Third nerve palsy in children is more frequently a congenital disorder than an acquired disorder, while acquired third nerve palsies appear more frequently in adults than in children.

CONGENITAL THIRD NERVE PALSY

Congenital third nerve palsy presents with varied degrees of extraocular involvement. The intraocular musculature is never affected in congenital third nerve palsy.

The degree of involvement of the levator muscle varies, but some function is usually retained.

Therefore, ptosis is variable in this form of third nerve palsy. The four extraocular muscles innervated by the third nerve are also affected in various degrees. However, there is usually some trace at least of weakness of the medial rectus muscle, the inferior rectus muscle, the superior rectus muscle, and the inferior oblique muscle. The fourth nerve is uninvolved and, consequently, the involved eye is exotropic and hypotropic (Fig 19-1). Therefore, the clinician should always suspect congenital third nerve palsy in an exotropic patient who has one low eye, intact pupillary and accommodation responses, and minimal ptosis of the involved eye with varied degrees of limitation of both elevation and depression in addition to diminished adduction. Many of these patients are able to develop single binocular vision and maintain a compensatory malposition of the head that allows the alignment of the eyes to serve this purpose. When the eyes are moved into a position where fusion is not possible, these patients experience diplopia if they have binocular vision with torticollis. Amblyopia of either eye may occur if the patient does not have binocular vision and does not maintain torticollis.

The cause of congenital third nerve palsy is unknown, but it is presumed to be due to a developmental defect either in the nuclear or motor fiber portion of the third nerve complex that innervates the levator muscle and the extraocular muscles. It is not an extremely rare motility disorder. The author has seen many patients having only unilateral involvement.

As in any third nerve palsy, the absence of adduction of the involved eye makes it difficult to determine the intactness of the ipsilateral fourth nerve. Clinically, the method used to investigate this question is to observe the crypts of the iris while the involved eye remains in the abducted position, commanding the patient to look upward and downward. If the fourth nerve is intact, the iris markings reveal a conspicuous intorsion as infraduction is attempted and extorsion as supraduction of the involved eye is attempted (Fig 19-2).

The forced duction test is negative in third nerve palsy; this rules out any adhesive phenomenon that would limit the motility of the eye. The degree of involvement of the third nerve determines whether or not therapy is indicated. The involvement may be so minor and partial that no therapy is necessary or it may affect only the elevators of an eye and is, therefore, known as double elevator palsy. Double elevator palsy is usually rather complete, and it may also be associated with various degrees of ptosis (Fig 19-3). The ptosis may be only pseudoptosis because of the hypotropia and the

153

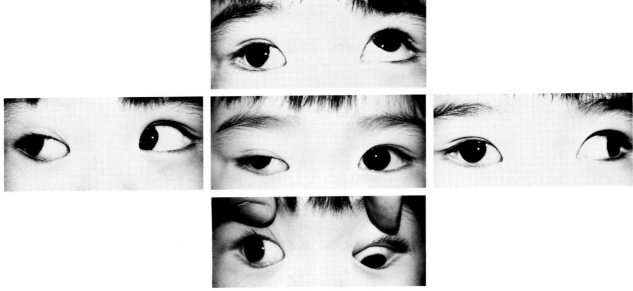

Fig 19-1. Congenital right third nerve palsy with exotropia, intact pupillary and accommodation responses, minimal ptosis, and diminished elevation, depression, and adduction of the involved eye.

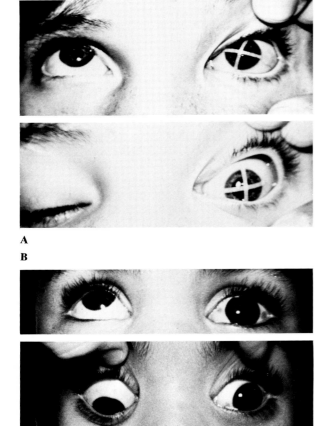

A

B

fact the lid position follows the eye position. Fixating with the hypotropic eye causes the complete disappearance of the pseudoptosis, however, there may be a small degree of bona fide ptosis in addition to the pseudoptosis. The traction test is normal in double elevator palsy. The treatment of double elevator palsy is to transposition the insertions of the horizontal rectus muscles, placing the new insertions immediately adjacent to the insertion of the superior rectus muscle (Fig 19-4). This does not produce normal elevation beyond the midline level, but it renders considerable improvement in, if not total elimination of, the hypotropia caused by this disorder.

Complete congenital third nerve involvement requires surgery for the exotropia, hypotropia and ptosis. The hypotropia is solved by disinserting the tendon of the superior oblique muscle from the globe which is tight and contracted. Maximal recession of the lateral rectus and resection of the medial rectus may be sufficient to satisfactorily reposition the involved eye in the horizontal plane. However, if this is inadequate, removal of the superior oblique tendon from the trochlea, severing the reflected tendon of the superior oblique muscle from the muscular portion and attaching the superior oblique muscle to the sclera at the insertion of the medial rectus muscle, offers excellent correc-

Fig 19-2. Intact fourth cranial nerve in third nerve palsy. **A.** Litmus paper marker on cornea. **B.** Pigmented scleral spots demonstrate intorsion as depression is attempted.

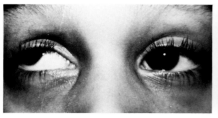
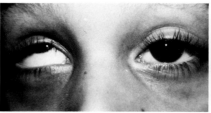
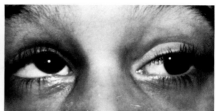
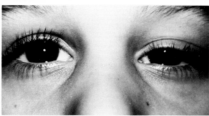

Fig 19-3. Double elevator palsy.

Fig 19-4. Transposition of the insertions of the horizontal rectus muscles superiorly for treatment of double elevator palsy. (Helveston, C. V. Mosby).

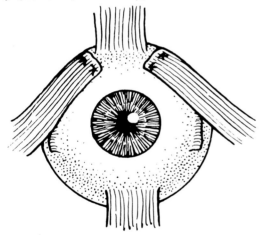

tion of the horizontal defect created by the third nerve palsy in the primary position. This does not create normal adduction of the involved eye. However, following the transposition of the superior oblique muscle when the patient depresses the involved eye, it adducts. A frontalis suspension of the ptotic lid is the indicated procedure for the associated ptosis. A synthetic material, eg, 4-0 Supramid, is ideal because if the cornea cannot tolerate the relatively dry state after the lid is elevated the synthetic sutures can easily be removed and the cornea is not permanently harmed. The surgeon should be aware of the absence of Bell's phenomenon in these patients and be alert to the postoperative corneal problems associated with this deficiency.

ACQUIRED THIRD NERVE PALSY

Acquired third nerve palsy may be partial or complete and may involve only the extraocular muscles or both intraocular and extraocular muscles. The pupil is usually spared in third nerve palsy associated with diabetes.

Acquired third nerve palsy usually occurs rather precipitously with maximal involvement. Within days or weeks, there may be an indication of restoration of third nerve function manifest by only partial involvement. Recovery is usually complete by six months following onset, and, consequently, no judgement should be rendered regarding the necessity of treatment until after the six-month interval. Many times the palsy is the result of relatively serious intracranial involvement, and this may determine whether or not therapy is indicated. The causes can be classified as follows:

  I. Brainstem Lesion
    A. Benedikt's syndrome manifest by homolateral third nerve paralysis and contralateral intention tremor
    B. Weber's syndrome manifest by homolateral third nerve paralysis and contralateral hemiplegia
 II. Inflammatory Conditions
    A. Meningitis
    B. Encephalitis
    C. Polyneuritis from toxins such as alcohol, lead, arsenic, and carbon monoxide, and from diabetes
    D. Herpes zoster
III. Vascular lesions (aneurysms)
IV. Tumors
 V. Demyelinating diseases
VI. Trauma

Treatment involves relief of the patient's diplopia which usually is not a problem in complete third nerve paralysis because of the associated ptosis covering the pupil. However, in partial involvement the lid may sufficiently clear the pupillary space so that diplopia is a problem. Occlusion therapy is the best solution for the patient's diplopia. The patient usually wishes to have the involved eye occluded rather than the uninvolved eye. Surgery is indicated for the strabismus and ptosis if the patient's general condition permits it and if a significant residual paralysis is present six months after onset of the third nerve palsy. The surgery described for congenital third nerve palsy is also applicable for acquired third nerve palsy.

FOURTH NERVE PALSY

The commonest cause of an isolated cyclovertical muscle palsy is involvement of the trochlear nerve. However, palsy of the superior oblique muscle must be differentiated from palsy of the other cyclovertical muscles which if paretic manifest a combined cyclovertical phoria or tropia. Each of the muscles that move the eye in a vertical plane about the X axis of Fick, including the superior oblique muscle, also renders a torsional movement about the Y axis of Fick.

The nature of the eye movement produced by contraction of a cyclovertical muscle depends on the horizontal position of the eye. In abduction, the vertical rectus muscles move the eye in the vertical plane and the oblique muscles in the torsional plane. In adduction, the vertical rectus muscles act torsionally, and the oblique muscles act vertically. Both the vertical rectus muscles and the oblique muscles deliver a combined vertical and torsional action in the primary position. The vertical actions and the cycloactions of the eight cyclovertical muscles in the primary position, dextroversion, and levoversion are shown in Figure 19-5. However, the action of the vertical rectus muscles is somewhat more vertical than torsional, whereas, the action of the oblique muscles is more torsional than vertical. Therefore, weakness of a single cyclovertical muscle is characterized by vertical and torsional deviation in the primary position. The torsional deviation increases on lateral gaze to one side, while the vertical deviation increases on opposite lateral gaze. For example, since the left superior oblique muscle is a depressor and intortor, weakness of this muscle results in left hypertropia that increases on right gaze and excyclotropia that increases on left gaze.

The diplopia seen by patients with fourth nerve palsy is a combined vertical and torsional set of images projected from the object of regard. The superior pole of the low image seen by the palsied eye is tilted inward as compared with the superior pole of the high image seen by the normal eye. By sending inhibitory innervation to the palsied muscle, the diplopia disappears. Since the superior oblique muscle is a depressor and intortor muscle, its tone is diminished by upgaze and by tilting the

Fig 19-5. Vertical and torsional actions of the cyclovertical acting muscles. (From Parks MM: Arch Ophthalmol 60:1027, 1958.)

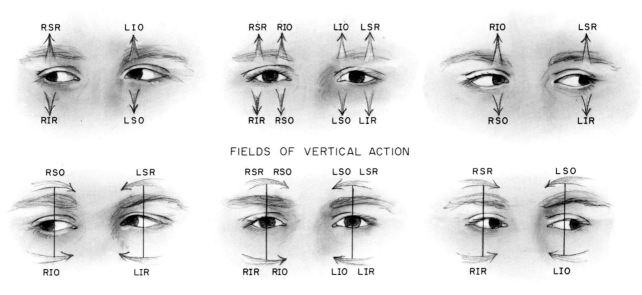

FIELDS OF VERTICAL ACTION

FIELDS OF CYCLO ACTION

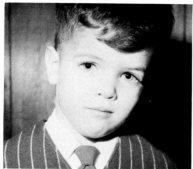

Fig 19-6. Left fourth nerve palsy with compensatory head posture, secondary overacting left inferior oblique muscle, and positive Bielschowsky head tilt test finding.

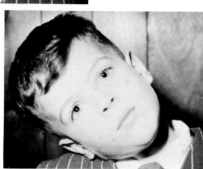
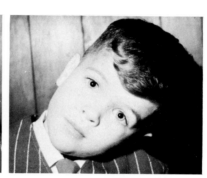

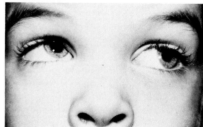

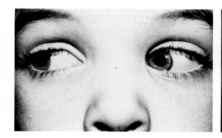
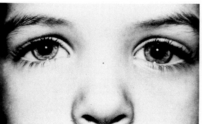
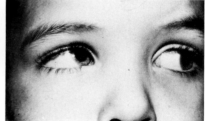

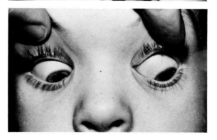

Patient's Right　　　　　　　　　　　　　*Patient's Left*

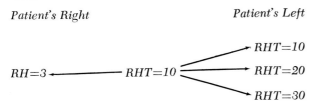

Fig 19-7. Cardinal field measurements in right fourth nerve palsy soon after onset.

Fig 19-8. Cardinal field measurements in right fourth nerve palsy late after onset.

Patient's Right　　　　　　　　　　　　　*Patient's Left*

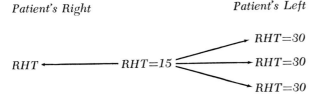

head to the shoulder opposite the palsied muscle which extorts this eye. The typical ocular torticollis noted in patients with fourth nerve palsy is chin depression and head tilt, as depicted in Figure 19-6.

Soon after onset of the fourth nerve palsy, the cardinal field test reveals the disorder since the hypertropia is maximal in the vertical field of action of the superior oblique muscle (Fig 19-7). However, as the palsy continues for many months, contracture of the ipsilateral inferior oblique muscle begins to manifest itself by eliminating the early cardinal field finding. On the side in which the vertical deviation of the eyes is maximal, the hypertropia measures the same in upgaze and downgaze, ie, the hypertropia becomes concomitant (Fig 19-8). Hence, vertical concomitance requires that some test other than cardinal field measurements be done to correctly diagnose the palsied cyclovertical muscle.

With vertical concomitance established, another sign of contracture of the direct antagonist inferior oblique muscle is the overelevation of the adducted palsied eye (secondary overaction of inferior oblique muscle, as described in the chapter entitled Oblique Muscle Dysfunctions).

By having the patient move the eyes into the cardinal fields, one can easily misdiagnose left superior rectus muscle palsy instead of correctly diagnosing right superior oblique muscle palsy and vice versa. The misdiagnosis occurs so frequently that it has received the auspicious name of inhibitional palsy of the contralateral antagonist. During cardinal field testing, as the patient fixates with the eye that is innervated by the palsied fourth nerve,

the underelevation of the abducted opposite eye is conspicuous to the examiner, who may be inclined to attribute this condition to palsy of the superior rectus muscle of the sound eye. This error in diagnosis is less apt to happen while the patient fixates with the sound eye because it makes the full movement in elevation and abduction, but fixating with the palsied eye makes the less than normal elevation in abduction of the sound eye obvious. This apparent deficiency in the function of the sound eye in this particular cardinal field is due to the less than usual innervation being dispatched to the inferior oblique muscle of the fixating palsied eye to drive against the atonic palsied superior oblique muscle in order to continue pursuit of an elevating adducting target. By the law of Herring, equal innervation is dispatched to yoke muscles, resulting in deficient innervation to drive the sound eye upward against the normal tone in its inferior rectus muscle. The terms "yoke" and "contralateral agonist" are synonymous terms for the same muscle. Both an agonist (palsied muscle) and a contralateral agonist (yoke to the palsied muscle) have antagonists (direct and contralateral). The superior rectus muscle of the sound eye is the contralateral antagonist to the palsied muscle. Since the mistaken diagnosis of palsy of the superior rectus muscle of the opposite eye in a patient with fourth nerve palsy is due to an inhibition of the normal innervation sent to carry out its normal function, the misdiagnosis is attributable to an inhibitional palsy of the contralateral antagonist, not to a bona fide palsy of an agonist.

To prevent erroneous diagnosis of fourth nerve palsy, the Bielschowsky head tilt test should always be done and the measurements recorded since contracture of the direct antagonist of the ipsilateral palsied muscle does not influence the findings.

To logically evaluate any isolated cyclovertical muscle palsy, including fourth nerve palsy, the accumulation of three separate pieces of information followed by three separate reasoning steps invariably provides an accurate diagnosis. The clinician should develop a policy of orderly applying three separate steps known as the 3 Step Test (1) which follows:

I. Step 1. Determining whether there is right hypertropia or left hypertropia in the primary position eliminates four of the eight cyclovertical muscles as being at fault. For example, right hypertropia signifies there is a
　A. Weak right depressor
　　1. Right inferior rectus
　　2. Right superior oblique
　B. Weak left elevator

1. Left superior rectus
2. Left inferior oblique

II. Step 2. Determining whether the vertical deviation increases on right or left gaze eliminates one of the two possible faulty muscles in each eye. For example:

A. Right hypertropia increases in left gaze, indicating either that the
   1. Right superior oblique is weak
   2. Left superior rectus is weak

B. At this point, the two possible faulty muscles are always either intortors or extortors. Never is one muscle an intortor and the other an extortor.

III. Step 3. The Bielschowsky head tilt test accurately differentiates which of the two muscles from the preceding step is at fault, for example, the right superior oblique or the left superior rectus.

The utricular reflex is stimulated by tilting the head. Tilting to the right causes the intortors of the right eye and the extortors of the left eye to contract, while the opposite combination contracts on tilting to the left. However, since the eyes remain in the primary position with reference to the skull, despite the change of the head position in the field of gravity, the contracting cyclovertical muscles render a combined torsional and vertical action. The two intortors or the two extortors of each eye that contract in response to head tilt have opposite vertical actions: one is an elevator and the other is a depressor. Normally, the opposite vertical actions cancel each other, while their identical torsional actions are additive; therefore, the eye remains on the same level in the vertical plane but cycloverts accordingly (Fig 19-9). This physiologic feature is the source of Step 3, as illustrated in Figure 19-10, depicting a palsied right intortor that is stimulated on right head tilt with its weak depressor action unable to offset the elevator action of its normal fellow intortor. Consequently, an increase of right hypertropia, on right head tilt and a decrease on left tilt diagnoses the right superior oblique as the palsied muscle. An increase of right hypertropia on left head tilt and a decrease on right head tilt diagnoses the left superior rectus as the palsied muscle.

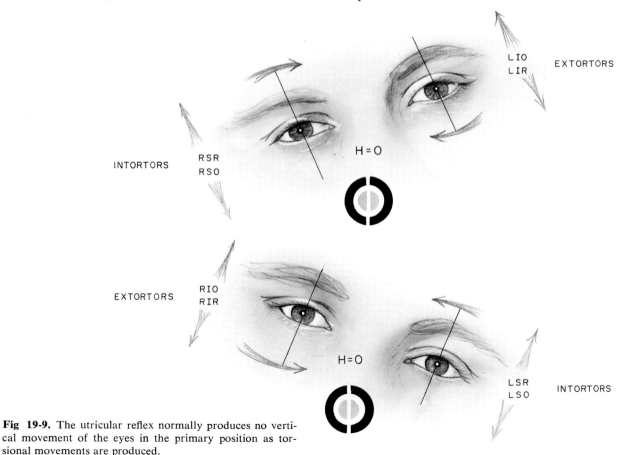

Fig 19-9. The utricular reflex normally produces no vertical movement of the eyes in the primary position as torsional movements are produced.

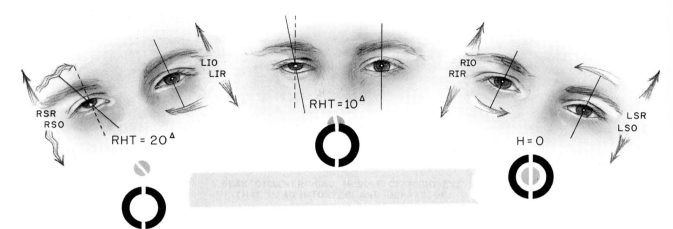

Fig 19-10. The utricular reflex produces an increase of right hyperdeviation on right head tilt and a reduction on left head tilt in right superior oblique muscle palsy.

Trochlear nerve palsies may be unilateral or bilateral; if they are bilateral, the involvement may be minimal on one side and maximal on the other. The minimally involved side may be masked entirely by the maximally involved eye until surgical therapy is performed to eliminate the motility defect and only then is it truly apparent that there must be different degrees of bilateral involvement. If bilateral involvement can be detected, there is right hypertropia in left gaze and left hypertropia in right gaze; the right hypertropia increases as the patient's head is tilted on the right shoulder and the left hypertropia increases with the head tilted to the left shoulder. There is also greater excyclotropia (10° or more) in bilateral involvement than in unilateral involvement.

The cause of congenital trochlear nerve palsy is a defect in the nucleus or motor portion of the nerve; a defect in the motor nerve occurs either intramedullarly or extramedullarly. The commonest cause of acquired fourth nerve palsy is closed head trauma. Intracranial tumors and aneurysms also account for the diagnosis in some patients. Displacement of the trochlea as a result of surgery on or trauma to the orbit is another cause.

The management of congenital fourth nerve palsy attracts clinical attention by six months of age because of either an obvious vertical strabismus or torticollis or both. Surgery on the cyclovertical muscle is indicated as soon as possible, even prior to 1 year of age if the surgeon is confident of his findings. Early surgery to decrease the obstacles to fusion offers the best chance of developing or maintaining binocular vision, and it is the only rational means of preventing the permanent musculoskeletal changes of torticollis, facial asymmetry, and scoliosis. The facial asymmetry in long-standing torticollis present during childhood is manifest by a shallow atrophied face on the low side; it is possibly due to reduced carotid artery blood flow as a result of pinching of the vessel, deviation of the nose toward the low side (possibly due to the effect of gravity), and a slanted mouth as though it were trying to assume a horizontal orientation.

Treatment of acquired fourth nerve palsy during the first six months is usually simply waiting to determine the degree of spontaneous recovery. After six months from onset, specific surgical correction of the acquired strabismus should be undertaken. Unless the hypertropia exceeds 20Δ in the primary position, only one muscle should be operated on at a time, and the degree of improvement should be studied over a three-month period prior to deciding whether or not further surgery is indicated.

The objective is to simultaneously improve the cyclodeviations and vertical deviations. This can only be achieved by operating on the following four of the eight cyclovertical muscles:

1. Agonist (paretic muscle)
2. Direct antagonist
3. Contralateral agonist (yoke)
4. Contralateral antagonist (direct antagonist of yoke)

If contracture of the direct antagonist is present, as manifested by its obvious overaction, and the vertical tropia is concomitant for upgaze and downgaze with the side of the vertical field of action of the palsied muscle, weakening the direct antagonist should be the first procedure. Otherwise, ie, in the absence of obvious contracture, one may weaken the yoke of the palsied muscle or tuck the palsied muscle as the first procedure. In general, the longer the duration of the strabismus the greater the likelihood of contracture of the direct antagonist.

Tightening of the palsied muscle does not make it normal. Mechanical improvement is obtained in the primary position, but there is still deficiency in the field of action of the paretic muscle. If the tuck is performed, it should be performed temporal to the superior rectus muscle. Performing the tuck at this site diminishes the restriction of elevation in adduction (simulated Brown's syndrome) but not entirely; the restricted elevation usually gradually improves. Therefore, some surgeons are less than enthusiastic about tucking the paretic superior oblique tendon unless further surgery is required after the yoke has been recessed.

The quantity of tendon tucked is 10 mm or more, depending on how easily it stretches out on the instrument used for tucking. Recessions of the inferior oblique muscle are usually 10 mm; if the overaction is extremely marked, recession may be increased to 14 mm. Recessions of the inferior rectus muscle range between 3 and 4 mm; if the vertical deviation in the primary position is 10Δ or more, the maximum recession is performed. Maximum recession causes approximately 1 mm of sclera to show peripheral to the 6-o'clock limbus position.

There are many exceptions to the above recommendation of which muscle should be operated on

first; the most notable exception is a patient having minimal palsy of the superior oblique muscle with no direct antagonist contracture. Tucking the superior oblique tendon yields greater benefit in this patient than in a patient with maximal paralysis of the superior oblique muscle.

Patients with bilateral fourth nerve palsy require bilateral surgery graded to the difference in the degree of palsy that exists between the two eyes.

SIXTH NERVE PALSY

Sixth nerve palsy causes esotropia in the primary position, which if unilateral increases on gaze direction toward the involved muscle. Continuation of binocular vision is usually possible by maintaining the eyes in the lateral gaze position away from the palsied eye; this results in a compensatory horizontal face position toward the palsied eye (Fig 19-11). Rapid forced dextroversion and levoversion movements reveal the slow floating abduction saccades of the palsied lateral rectus muscle as compared with the brisk normal rapid saccades of the other three horizontal rectus muscles.

The clinical courses of congenital and acquired sixth nerve palsies are dissimilar in one respect. Patients with congenital palsy and those with recently acquired palsy manifest greater primary position esotropia when they attempt to fixate with the palsied eye (secondary deviation) and lesser deviation when they fixate with the sound eye (primary deviation), thus the axiom "secondary deviation exceeds primary deviation." This charac-

Fig 19-11. Compensatory face turn in lateral rectus muscle palsy.

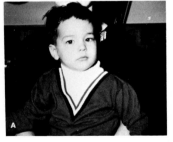

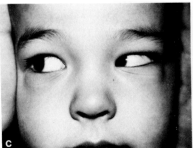
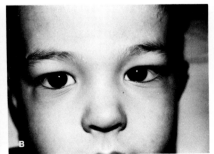
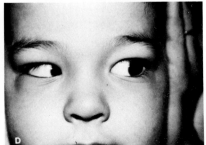

teristic gradually disappears during the first few months after the onset of an acquired lateral rectus muscle palsy due to contracture of the ipsilateral medial rectus muscle antagonist and hypertrophy of the yoke medial rectus muscle in the contralateral eye. This change occurs rapidly in young children whose acquired sixth nerve palsy eventually presents as a concomitant esotropia; it has no resemblance to the original nonconcomitant esotropia that suddenly appeared two to three months earlier. However, in all age-groups, persistent sixth nerve palsy that initially manifests as secondary deviation exceeding primary deviation eventually presents as identical primary position esotropia regardless of which eye is fixating, except in the patients who have congenital sixth nerve palsy.

By covering the sound eye, encouraging the palsied eye to maximally abduct while attempting fixation of an object in the field of action of the palsied muscle, and then covering both eyes, past pointing reveals that the patient with sixth nerve palsy points beyond the object as he attempts to localize it by memory. The effort involved in attempting to abduct the palsied eye influences the psycho-optic reflex, giving the impression that the object was farther to the side than it actually was.

CONGENITAL SIXTH NERVE PALSY

Congenital palsy of the sixth nerve is rare, although literature on the subject suggests otherwise. Much of the literature suggests that the diagnosis is confused with congenital esotropia, Duane's retraction syndrome, and Möbius' syndrome. Birth trauma has been proposed as a major cause of this diagnosis, but this is questionable. There are probably some patients with hypoplasia of the abducens motor nucleus, or an anomaly within the motor nerve fibers, but these are few. Also, some lateral rectus muscles have been described as absent or hypoplastic, but overall the frequency of this description is low. Yet, misdiagnosis of congenital sixth nerve palsy by confusing it with congenital esotropia, Duane's retraction syndrome, and Möbius' syndrome has been and continues to be frequent.

ACQUIRED SIXTH NERVE PALSY

Because of the long intracranial course, angulated over the petrous tip of the temporal bone, and the absence of any slack in the course between the brainstem and the dura entry, the sixth nerve is vulnerable to increased intracranial pressure, trauma to the cranial floor, meningeal edema, inflammation in the base of the skull, and any displacement of the brainstem. It also shares with the other cranial nerves the sensitivities to toxic substances, the affliction with acute demyelinating diseases, and exposure to attack by viruses. Tumors and aneurysms are the relatively common causes of displacement of the brainstem and the abducens nerve. Cerebral tumors displace the brainstem downward, cerebellar tumors displace it forward, anterior infratentorial tumors push the brainstem backward, cerebellopontine angle tumors push it laterally, and a nasopharyngeal tumor can make pressure from below. Intramedullary lesions in the pons can cause ipsilateral sixth nerve palsy and contralateral hemiplegia (Millard-Gubler syndrome) or contralateral intention tremor. Thrombosis in the posterior portion of the basilar artery may cause sixth nerve palsy. (Thrombosis in the anterior basilar artery usually causes third nerve palsy.) Neuritis of the sixth nerve occurs in the presence of diabetes, lead and arsenic poisoning, diphtheria and tetanus toxins, and in thiamine deficiency. A host of viruses have been implicated in sixth nerve palsy, including herpes zoster, anterior poliomyelitis, encephalitis lethargica, influenza, and typhus. Meningeal irritations following lumbar puncture, spinal anesthesia, and spinal pantopaque myelography plus meningitis are other causes of sixth nerve palsy.

A special form of meningeal irritation and edema resulting from middle ear infection and causing sixth nerve palsy deserves special comment. Middle ear infection associated with petrositis and edema of its dura or possibly thrombosis in the contiguous venous sinuses pinches the sixth nerve against the petrosphenoidal ligament (Gruber's ligament) as it passes between it and the dura (Dorello's canal), causing Gradenigo's syndrome. Young children are prone to this disorder, which is associated with respiratory infection, elevated temperature, and, frequently, facial pain. The frequency of repeated episodes of palsy is high; the duration is usually brief because of the effectiveness of antibiotics, and improvement is obvious within three to six weeks. If the palsy persists, contracture of the medial rectus muscle occurs, and a permanent concomitant esotropia replaces the nonconcomitant esotropia that was originally controlled with compensatory head posture.

Management of unilateral sixth nerve palsy is symptomatic during the first few months after onset. The homonoymous diplopia in many patients is controlled by compensatory head posture and requires no treatment. Some patients who are unable to control the diplopia are not sufficiently disturbed to desire relief obtainable by occluding one eye; however, some are very annoyed and find relief with occlusion. Young children who do not control the esotropia with compensatory head posture should receive alternate occlusion (the right eye one day and the left eye the following day) to prevent development of amblyopia, suppression, and abnormal retinal correspondence. Fresnel prism spectacles with sufficient base-out power may be used in lieu of occulsion. Occluding the sound eye or placing a base-out prism before it has been claimed by some to prevent contracture of the ipsilateral direct antagonist (medial rectus muscle) to the paretic muscle, but this claim has not been documented.

Recovery from the sixth nerve palsy can usually be observed by three months after onset. If improvement does not occur within the first six months, surgery to correct the primary position esotropia should be undertaken. The surgery should include maximal recession of the ipsilateral medial rectus muscle since usually there is obvious contracture by this time. If sufficient primary position esotropia is present, recessing the contralateral medial rectus muscle may also be helpful, provided that the traction test for passive abduction of the palsied eye is normal following the recession of its medial rectus muscle. Resection of the paretic lateral rectus muscle provides some mechanical benefit in eliminating persistent primary position esotropia and is particularly helpful if the traction test for passive abduction is still positive following recession of the medial rectus muscle of the palsied eye. However, the abduction deficiency is not corrected by resection of the lateral rectus muscle, although it causes a restriction of adduction. Other procedures have their exponents: some claim great success with the Hummelsheim operation while others prefer the Jensen operation, as illustrated in Figure 19-12. In the Hummelsheim operation, the lateral halves of the superior and inferior rectus muscles are transpositioned to the superior and inferior poles of the scleral insertions of the lateral rectus muscle, and the medial rectus muscle is recessed; all of the surgery is performed on the involved eye. The same principle is used in the Jensen operation, but it is accomplished by securing together, with nonabsorbable sutures, loops of the temporal halves of the superior and inferior rectus muscles, respectively, to the superior and inferior loops of the halved lateral rectus muscle at approximately 12 mm back from their scleral insertions. The end result of the two procedures is comparable, but the blood supply to the anterior

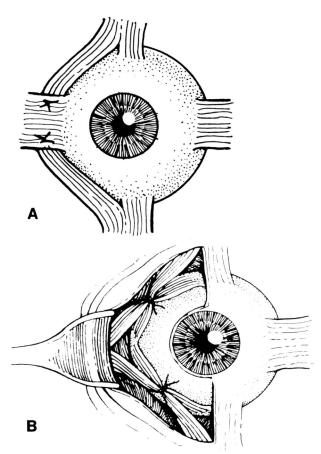

Fig 19-12. A. Hummelsheim operation. **B.** Jensen operation.

segment of the globe is probably compromised less by the Jensen procedure.

The argument continues about the best method to overcome the esotropia, but probably the most important surgical principle that must be obeyed in attempting to correct nonconcomitant esotropia associated with sixth nerve palsy is to do whatever is necessary to overcome the traction that keeps the palsied eye turned inward. Recessing the contractured direct antagonist muscle is invariably the first procedure that must be done in satisfying this principle. Resection of the palsied lateral rectus muscle, a Hummelsheim procedure, or a Jensen procedure are secondary procedures that offer an abducting pull on the palsied eye and further counter the adducting traction of the direct antagonist; these should be added to the medial rectus muscle recession if necessary. Resection of the palsied lateral rectus muscle is probably the most logical and simple of the secondary surgical procedures. If still further surgery is required to get the palsied eye into the straight ahead position, the Jensen procedure is probably the least traumatic procedure.

REFERENCE

1. Parks MM: Isolated cyclovertical muscle palsy. Arch Ophthalmol 60:1027, 1958

20

Ophthalmoplegic Syndromes and Trauma

DUANE'S RETRACTION SYNDROME

Prior to Duane's description in 1905, this syndrome was described by Stilling in 1887 and Turk in 1896 and, consequently, is named more correctly the Stilling-Turk-Duane syndrome. Duane emphasized that retraction of the adducted involved globe is an essential clinical feature of this syndrome, and since this feature is so diagnostic, common usage of the designation Duane's retraction syndrome is deeply entrenched and should be continued.

The clinical presentation of Duane's retraction syndrome is varied. Invariably, in addition to retraction of the adducted globe, the patient exhibits a defect in horizontal motility. Also, a vertical motility defect frequently occurs in adduction. Various contributors to the literature have categorized Duane's syndrome (1, 2) into subtypes, but this is not too helpful since one type merges with another. Furthermore, the various subclassifications are confusing since some are based on clinical findings while others are based on electromyographic findings. The most characteristic clinical presentation of Duane's syndrome is an absence of abduction of an eye with some degree of restricted adduction and retraction while attempting to adduct (Fig 20-1). The retraction is variable: it is conspicuous in some but minimal in others. Also, either an upshooting or downshooting, or both, of the adducted eye frequently occurs, particularly as the adducting eye begins to move in the oblique position

of up and in or down and in. This overshoot simulates overaction of the inferior and superior oblique muscles. Occasionally, the upshoot or downshoot is so marked that the cornea is driven completely out of the palpebral fissure, hiding it behind the upper or lower lid. Some patients manifest only the upshoot and a few only the downshoot, but the majority of the patients have various degrees of both vertical abnormalities.

Duane's retraction syndrome may be bilateral, and, although it most commonly involves the left eye, it may involve only the right eye. Duane's retraction syndrome occurs more frequently in females than in males. Two excellent independent statistical studies have confirmed these facts. Kirkham (3) determined that 1 percent of the people with strabismus have Duane's retraction syndrome. In his study of 100 patients, 65 were female. The left eye was involved in 60 percent of the patients, the right eye in 22 percent, and there was bilateral involvement in 18 percent. In reporting on 186 patients with Duane's syndrome, Pfaffenbach, Cross, and Kearns (4) found that 57 percent of the patients were female; the left eye was involved in 60 percent of the patients, the right eye in 21 percent, and bilateral involvement in 19 percent.

Duane's retraction syndrome is frequently associated with the Klippel-Feil anomaly; it occurred in 4 percent of the patients from Kirkham's series and in 3 percent of the patients from Pfaffenbach, Cross, and Kearns' series. Congenital labyrinthine deafness is also often associated with this syndrome; 11 percent of Kirkham's patients and 7.5 percent of Pfaffenbach, Cross, and Kearns' series manifested this association. Duane's retraction syndrome, the Klippel-Feil anomaly, and congenital labyrinthine deafness constitute the syndrome of Wildervanck (5). The epibulbar dermoids and preauricular skin tags comprising Goldenhar's syndrome occur more frequently in patients with Duane's syndrome than in unaffected people. The majority of patients with Duane's syndrome seem to be sporadic cases; however, it has been reported by some and observed by this author in three instances as a dominant inherited defect.

The majority of patients with Duane's syndrome have straight eyes in the primary position, at least during infancy and childhood. The minority gradually develop an increasing esodeviation in the primary position that is offset by the restricted adduction of the involved eye. These patients find it possible to continue their normal binocular status; they adopt a compensatory turn of the head toward the side of the involved eye, thus offsetting the lateral gaze position that the eyes must assume in

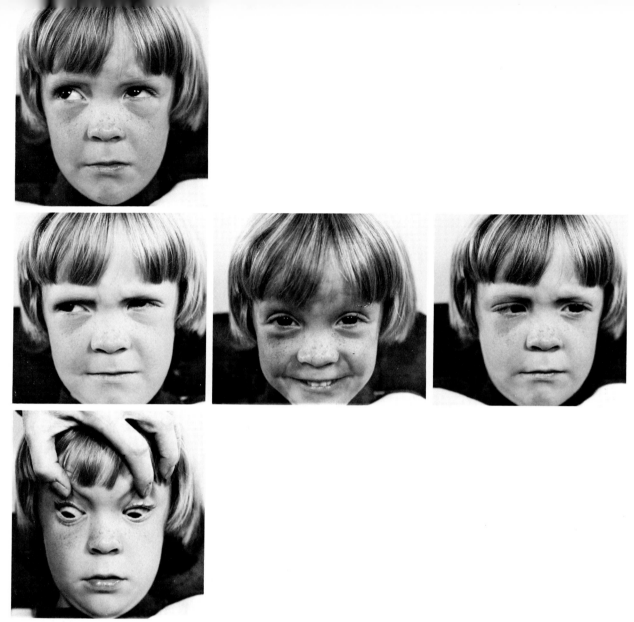

Fig 20-1. Duane's retraction syndrome, left eye.

order to continue normal binocular vision. Usually, the quantity of abduction that the involved eye is capable of is nil; in some the eye cannot be abducted even to the zero straight ahead position. Yet, a few patients with Duane's syndrome can abduct the involved eye many degrees; they may have severe restriction of adduction in this eye with retraction on abduction, rather than abduction. This latter variety is designated as "inverse Duane's retraction syndrome" by many.

Until the advent of electromyography · (6), Duane's retraction syndrome was attributed to replacement of the normal contractile substance within the lateral rectus muscle with fibrous tissue. This thesis supposedly explained the abduction deficiency, the restricted adduction, the retraction, and the frequency encountered upshoot and downshoot of the adducting eye. Biopsy specimens of the lateral rectus muscle often revealed an increase in fibrous tissue, possibly resulting from a change that occurs secondary to abnormal innervation. The more recent electromyographic evidence is overwhelming that primarily the cause of this disorder is paradoxic innervation. Electromyograms of the lateral rectus muscle usually show a silent tracing on abduction and firing on adduction. The co-contraction of the horizontal rectus muscles on adduction causes the retraction of the globe (7). The various degrees of the paradoxic innervation abnormality determine whether or not any abduction of the involved eye occurs; the degree of retraction of the eye on adduction is also determined. Furthermore, secondary anatomic changes may occur in the abnormally innervated lateral and medial rectus muscles, producing the positive traction test finding and the gradual esodeviation change that occurs in the primary position of some patients.

Surgery for Duane's syndrome is contraindicated, since it cannot correct the anomalous innervation, unless the patient has adopted an unsightly compensatory head posture. Most patients eventually learn to mask the bad appearance caused by their motility defect by turning the head rather than the eyes to view in lateral gaze, thus revealing their noncomitant esotropia on side gaze only when making a sudden lateral gaze movement when startled. However, surgery is indicated if a compensatory head posture develops to offset a primary position horizontal tropia. The purpose of the surgery is to restore the eyes to a parallel alignment in the primary position, making the unsightly compensatory face turn unnecessary. The prognosis is excellent, provided that the esoturned involved eye has been surgically brought out to the zero straight ahead position.

At surgery, the medial rectus muscle of the involved eye is almost invariably thick, hypertrophied, and taut, and the external capsule is often tightly adhered to rather than separated from Tenon's capsule by lax check ligaments. After the medial rectus muscle is freed from Tenon's capsule and disinserted, the positive traction test that manifested resistance to passive abduction is converted to negative. Patients receiving surgery for the compensatory head posture due to the esodeviated retracted eye require maximal recession of the medial rectus muscle. In addition to the recession, if the medial rectus is extremely tight, a Z tenotomy can be performed on this muscle at the same time that it is maximally recessed. Resection of the lateral rectus muscle should not be performed since an increase in the retraction of the globe follows this procedure. If retraction of the globe is marked and if there is extreme narrowing of the palpebral fissure on attempted adduction, the lateral rectus muscle can be recessed at the same time that the medial rectus muscle is weakened. Recessing the lateral rectus muscle does not augment the deficiency of abduction, but it improves the retraction of the globe that occurs on adduction. Whatever

surgery is performed to eliminate the primary position esodeviation in Duane's retraction syndrome also further aggravates the adduction weakness. Transposition of the muscles, which entails moving all or portions of the vertical rectus muscles temporally to assist the deficient pull power of the rectus muscle, with the intention of giving the patient abduction beyond the zero straight ahead position should not be considered because this causes further embarrassment of adduction. The minimal gain in abduction from such procedures as the Hummelsheim, Jensen (Fig 19-12), or total vertical rectus muscle temporal transpositions is unjustified when it is weighed against the significant adduction loss.

BROWN'S SYNDROME

The motility defect manifest by an inability to raise the adducted eye above the midhorizontal plane was first described by Brown (1, 8, 9). Less elevation restriction is usually apparent in the midline and even a smaller elevation deficiency is detectable in abduction. Slight downshoot of the adducting involved eye is often present although no overdepression, simulating overaction of the superior oblique muscle, occurs. A widening of the palpebral fissure on adduction is associated with this elevation restriction (Fig 20-2). Increasing exodeviation usually occurs as the eyes are moved upward in the midline.

Brown (10) has redefined this syndrome, recognizing that it is more complex than originally thought since it constitutes a spectrum of varying degrees and different causes. Brown initially reasoned that the simulated inferior oblique muscle palsy comprising this syndrome was due to an innervational deficit to this muscle, with secondary contracture of the anterior sheath of the superior oblique tendon. Electromyography proved this concept erroneous by invariably demonstrating normal innervation to the inferior oblique on attempted upgaze. However, Brown describes the true sheath syndrome as congenital, permanent, and invariably associated with a positive traction test manifested by inability to passively elevate the adducted involved eye. Most patients have no vertical misalignment in the primary position, but in some the involved eye is hypotropic and fusion occurs only in downgaze, causing a compensatory chin-up face posture. Incising or removing the tendon sheath has not produced good results in improving the compensatory head posture or in overcoming the primary position vertical tropia or the elevation deficiency of the adducted involved eye. These poor

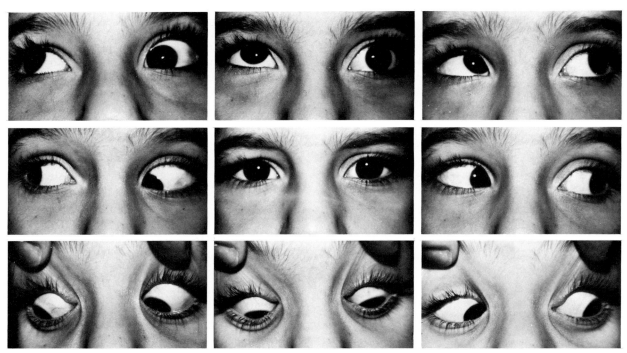

Fig 20-2. Brown's syndrome.

results have caused some doubt that the taut anterior sheath is the cause of this syndrome. Improvement has resulted from tenotomizing the superior oblique tendon, but this procedure has in turn produced a new problem, ie, palsy of the tenotomized superior oblique muscle associated with the opposite vertical tropia in downgaze that is offset with torticollis. Undoubtedly, a taut superior oblique tendon is the cause of this syndrome in many patients but certainly not in all patients. Some of the patients with this syndrome who have been explored surgically by the author have a normally limp superior oblique tendon and sheath, and it is inconceivable that either the tendon or the sheath could interfere with elevating the adducted eye. All of the other extraocular muscles were explored surgically for other possible causes of the motility defect, but nothing was found; however, results of the positive traction test seem to suggest that the cause of restricted motility is posterior to the globe.

The patient who has the compensatory head posture and an unequivocal positive traction test presents a difficult problem to the surgeon, particularly if the superior oblique tendon is normally limp. To improve this patient's compensatory head posture and the vertical tropia in the primary position, surgery on the other eye is required, eg,

recession of the contralateral superior rectus muscle and/or resection of the contralateral inferior rectus muscle. Nothing can be accomplished by resecting or plicating the ipsilateral inferior oblique muscle or by advancing its insertion since it is impossible to elevate the eye by the traction test. Scott and Knapp (11) removed the sheath tissue from around the superior oblique tendon and sutured the eye with coarse nonabsorbable material that was passed through the horizontal rectus muscles near their insertion to the nasal portion of the upper lid, fixing it in an upturned adducted position for several days. The results produced by this procedure have been equivocal and controversial.

A group of patients who manifest resistance to elevation in adduction and who on occasion can elevate the adducted involved eye are included in the spectrum of this motility defect. The elevation is abrupt and associated with an audible "snap" that both the examiner and the patient can palpate in the superior nasal orbit. Pressing the nasal orbital tissue with the index finger often assists the abrupt elevation of the involved eye as though whatever is restraining the movement is released by this pressure. This intermittent inability to elevate the adducted eye may be acquired at any age and also may eventually disappear. The traction test in this latter type of patient may be normal or at least less unequivocally abnormal than in the more severe variety of this syndrome. Brown considers these patients to have something other than the true sheath syndrome; hence, he describes them as having a simulated sheath syndrome. According to Brown, their motility disorder may be congenital; he attributes this to a thickened area in the superior oblique tendon posterior to the trochlea or some firm attachment between the posterior tendon and the posterior sheath, which interferes with the forward movement of the tendon through the trochlea. Brown considers the acquired simulated sheath syndrome to be secondary to an inflammatory process extending from the contiguous ethmoid cells to the posterior sheath and tendon. The author has operated on one patient who developed Brown's syndrome secondary to surgery for frontal sinusitis; at surgery the superior oblique tendon was found to be extremely taut and the tissue of Tenon's capsule covering the superior oblique tendon and superior rectus muscle was thick, opaque, and yellowish. The superior oblique tendon was as taut as the tendon encountered in 9 other patients who had a severe degree of congenital Brown's syndrome with manifest chin elevation and vertical strabismus in the primary position. Rheumatoid arthritis has been associated with this entity, and it is presumed that some nodule forms on the posterior tendon of the superior oblique muscle to account for the motility defect. Tucking of the superior oblique tendon also produces Brown's syndrome. An adherent phenomenon in either the superior or inferior nasal quadrant of the anterior orbit produces the same motility defect as found in Brown's syndrome.

The motility defect as described by Brown is a definite entity with many different causes. The cause of this defect in the majority of patients remains undetermined, but the sheath of the superior oblique tendon is probably blameless, although the tendon itself is undoubtedly short and taut in many of the patients. Therefore, Brown's syndrome is an appropriate designation for the disorder in these patients but sheath syndrome is probably inaccurate and misleading.

Similar to Duane's syndrome, no surgery is indicated in Brown's syndrome unless there is a need to improve the unsightly compensatory head posture that the patient adopts for the purpose of continuing binocular vision.

MÖBIUS' SYNDROME

The abnormal ocular motility involved in Möbius' syndrome is only a portion of this relatively extensive malady. The horizontal versions are congenitally absent in this syndrome. Congenital esotropia is often present, yet some patients are orthophoric in the primary position. A or V patterns are common in Möbius' syndrome, and if straight eyes can be achieved in either up or downgaze, a compensatory head posture is adopted to continue binocular vision.

Esotropia and inability to abduct the eyes are the usual reasons for the patient to be referred to the ophthalmologist. Horizontal versions are lacking, but vertical version and convergence are intact (Fig 20-3). Because of the inability to move the eyes horizontally in response to horizontal version stimulation, the patient may maintain fixation of the laterally moving target by voluntarily converging. Pupillary constriction and increasing accommodation occur as the voluntary convergence increases while visually tracking the target farther and farther into either right or left gaze.

Bilateral seventh cranial nerve palsy is manifest in the orbicularis muscles by the lower lids being lax, allowing the tears to pool between the lower lid and the bulbar conjunctiva. Forced closure of the lids may be inadequate to even approximate the upper and lower lid, but if they can be closed, the examiner can easily pry them apart (Fig 20-4). The seventh nerve palsy is further manifest by the expressionless smooth face, absent nasolabial folds, round mouth, and the inability to normally grin and wrinkle the forehead.

The most consistent associated defect encountered in Möbius' syndrome is palsy of the tongue which is manifest by an abnormal sucking reflex during infancy. The history provided by the parents indicates that the neonatal difficulty in maintaining the infant's weight occurred because of the feeding problem. The tongue palsy is also manifest in the abnormal phonation and the development of retarded speech. The terminal third of the tongue is atrophied, characterized by being furrowed, fissured, narrow, and pointed (Fig 20-5). Some degree of mental retardation is usual, and frequently there is an associated deafness. Osteologic defects are common in the form of supernumerary digits, syndactyly, brachydactyly, clubbed feet, rockerbottom feet, atrophy of the peroneal muscles, and a peculiar gait. Associated defects in the musculature of the neck and chest may be found.

The cause of the motility, facial, and tongue findings in Möbius' syndrome is aplasia of the nuclei of the abducens, facial, and glossopharyngeal nerves. The medial longitudinal fasciculi are probably also defective.

Since patients with Möbius' syndrome often have esotropia that was present at birth, they must be differentiated from those with the usual type of congenital esotropia. Although surgery for strabismus should be performed at a young age, as is

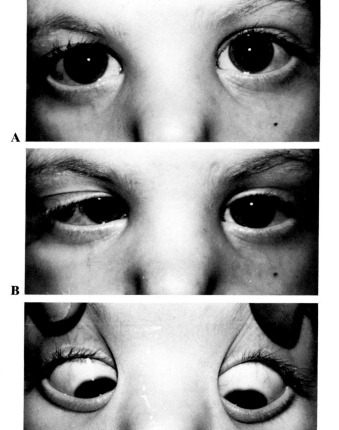

A

B

C

Fig 20-3. Möbius' syndrome. **A.** Primary position. **B.** Convergence. **C.** Downgaze.

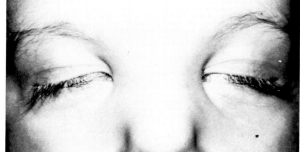

A

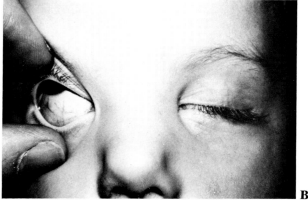

B

Fig 20-4. Möbius' syndrome. **A.** Forced closure of lids. **B.** Examiner prying lids apart.

Fig 20-5. Tongue in Möbius' syndrome.

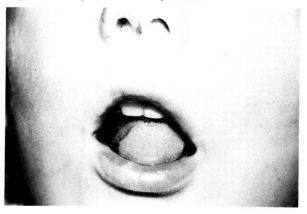

advocated for the primary type of congenital esotropia, invariably the traction tests and the character of the muscles encountered at surgery in patients with Möbius' syndrome are abnormal. The positive traction test shows passive resistance to both adduction and abduction while the vertical ductions are normal. The horizontal muscles are taut, thickened, fibrotic, and they resemble the medial rectus muscle usually found in the involved eye of Duane's syndrome.

FIBROSIS SYNDROMES

The tissue of the extraocular muscle is abnormal because of the replacement of the normal contractile substance with fibrous tissue, interfering with movement of the eye. The movement interference may result from either lack of pull power within the fibrotic muscle or resistance offered by the fibrotic muscle to its normally contracting antagonist. The latter has been speculated to produce retraction of the globe; this is the old thesis which is used to explain Duane's retraction syndrome. The fibrosis syndromes are extremely varied: they range from congenital to acquired, unilateral or bilateral, affecting all of the muscles of both eyes or only one muscle, and the degree of fibrosis of a muscle is total or partial.

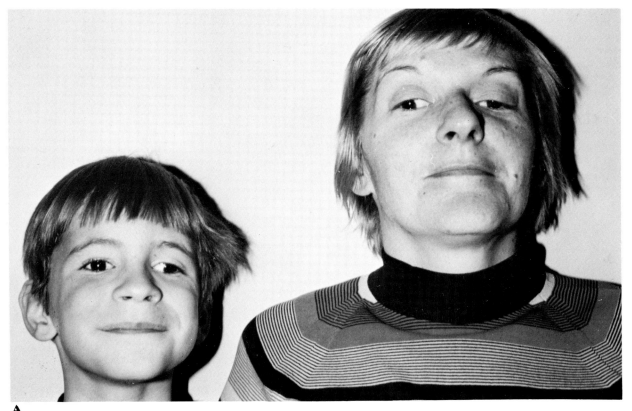

A

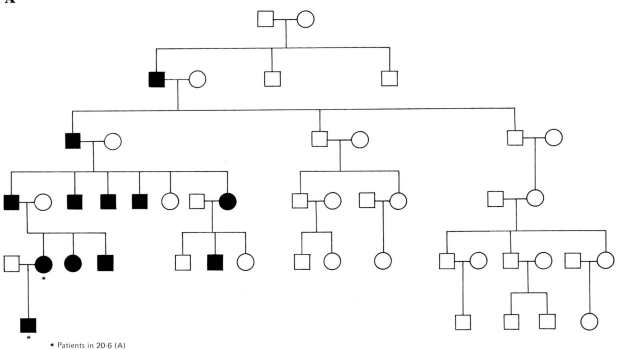

B

* Patients in 20-6 (A)

Fig 20-6. A. Generalized fibrosis syndrome. **B.** Autosomal dominant.

GENERALIZED FIBROSIS SYNDROME

All muscles, including the levator muscle, tend to be involved in this bilateral syndrome, although the muscles of one eye may be more involved than those of the other. Some muscles may be minimally fibrotic while others are maximally involved. The inferior rectus muscles are usually the most prone to maximal involvement, causing the eyes to be drawn downward and offering resistance to elevation in abduction and midline. Ptosis is associated with the motility defect in the eye. Horizontal movements of the eye may be limited to a few degrees in one or both directions or there may be no horizontal movement. Because of the down-turned fixed position of the globes, the patients usually adopt a chin-up position in order to centrally fixate straight ahead. This is a dominantly inherited condition affecting multiple family members (Fig 20-6).

The surgical approach to center these eyes and to improve the compensatory head posture must be unorthodox. Recessions of the inferior rectus muscles of 8 mm or more are required to allow the eyes to come to a relatively level position. Bilateral frontalis suspension surgery for the ptosis is the safest approach due to the absence of a Bell's phenomenon. If the corneas are unable to adjust to the relatively dry state following the surgery for the ptosis, the frontalis suspension permanent sutures can always be removed. Surgery for the ptosis can be combined with the recessions of the inferior rectus muscles.

CONGENITAL FIBROSIS OF THE INFERIOR RECTUS MUSCLE

Congenital fibrosis of the inferior rectus muscle is probably a variant of the generalized fibrosis syndrome, but only the inferior rectus muscle becomes involved because of its peculiar predilection for becoming fibrotic. The condition may be unilateral or bilateral, but if it is bilateral, it is usually asymmetric with greater involvement of one eye. Vertical strabismus is inevitable with this disorder, and if the patient maintains binocular vision, a compensatory chin-up posture is adopted.

Congenital fibrosis of the inferior rectus muscle must be differentiated from double elevator palsy in which the traction test is normal; however, with fibrosis of the inferior rectus muscle, it is impossible to passively elevate the eye. Surgical correction of this disorder requires maximal recession of the inferior rectus muscle. As soon as the inferior rectus muscle is disinserted, the traction test is converted to normal.

VERTICAL RETRACTION SYNDROME

Khodadoust and von Noorden (12) described a vertical retraction syndrome comprising inability to depress either eye while abducted and resistance offered to elevating either eye in abduction. In addition to the vertical duction limitation in each eye of two siblings, they describe the retraction of each eye during attempted depression while the eye is in the abducted position. One patient had exotropia on upgaze and the other patient had exotropia on downgaze, otherwise horizontal alignment in the primary position was satisfactory. These authors speculated that fibrosis of the vertical rectus muscles accounted for the retraction of the globe on downgaze. Presumably the fibrosis was confined principally to the superior rectus muscles. The traction test was positive in both patients for both upgaze and downgaze limitation.

STRABISMUS FIXUS

Strabismus fixus is a marked fixed position of either an in-turned or an out-turned eye or eyes. Tightness of the medial rectus muscle or muscles which are fibrous bands causes the eye or eyes to turn inward, and tightness of the lateral rectus muscle or muscles causes the widely fixed eye or eyes to turn outward. The eyes may be so firmly fixed in their far deviated horizontal position that it is impossible to horizontally displace them, either actively by the patient or passively by the traction test. These patients are benefited by tenotomy of the fibrous bands, but it is difficult to surgically gain access to them. Since this is a congenital disorder, these patients are devoid of any form of binocular vision and free of any diplopia. If the tenotomy permits the eyes to move around toward a straight position, allowing surrender of the severe adopted horizontal compensatory head posture required to see straight ahead, the patient is appreciative of both the visual and comfort gain.

THYROTOXICOSIS OPHTHALMOPLEGIA

The gross exophthalmos of thyrotoxicosis caused by the increase in the intraorbital tissue, mainly the muscles which are enlarged, reduces the motility of the eyes to practically zero. The elevation of the eye is particularly limited, and this probably leads to fibrosis of the inferior rectus muscles. Early in the disease, mucin is deposited in the extraocular muscles, causing edema because of its hydrophilic property. As the thyrotoxicosis is brought under control and as exophthalmos subsides, the muscles return to their normal size. However, fibrosis of the inferior rectus muscle may have developed, causing hypotropia as cicatrization occurs during the ensuing months. The traction test is positive, revealing inability to passively elevate the involved eye. Any one or several of the rectus muscles may be involved, but since the inferior rectus muscle has a predilection for becoming fibrotic, it is most frequently involved. A chin-up compensatory head posture is ordinarily used by these patients to see on the straight level or to fuse if the condition is unilateral.

After the condition stabilizes, an 8-mm recession of the fibrotic inferior rectus muscle or muscles is performed. This allows the eye or eyes to come to the straight level position. Although a limitation of upgaze persists, it is not disabling.

OPHTHALMOPLEGIAS

The ophthalmoplegias comprise a group of motility disorders associated with transient or permanent changes occurring at either the myoneural junction or within the muscle fiber.

PROGRESSIVE EXTERNAL OPHTHALMOPLEGIA

Progressive myopathy of the extraocular muscles is invariably bilateral, but it may affect one eye before the other. In the end stage, the condition is remarkably symmetric. It may be either sporadic or hereditary; if it is hereditary, it is usually autosomal dominant.

Acquired ptosis is usually the first sign of the disorder, and the other extraocular muscles may not reveal their condition until some years later. It often starts toward the latter part of the first decade of life or during adolescence, but it may be delayed until the first 20 or 30 years of life pass. The important feature of this disease is progression. The medial rectus muscle is the most frequently involved of the extraocular muscles, and if strabismus appears, exotropia is common. Elevation weakness usually appears before depression weakness, and this causes the patient to adopt a compensatory chin-up posture; however, as the condition progresses, the motility of the eyes eventually decreases to zero. The intraocular muscles of the eye are not involved.

Progressive external ophthalmoplegia is often associated with involvement of other muscle groups, particularly the sternomastoid muscles, the deltoid, and the trapezius. The related condition involving the various muscle groups of the body is hereditary progressive muscular dystrophy, and it may be difficult to separate these two disorders. However, it is not related to the hereditary chronic progressive myotonic dystrophy that most frequently affects the muscles of the upper portion of the body before progressing to the other skeletal muscles. The latter condition is associated with cataracts that are usually acquired in the latter part of the second decade of life, and it is also frequently associated with a retinal dystrophy.

The electromyogram is diagnostic for this condition which shows normal recruitment but low amplitude. Treatment entails supporting the lids either by crutch spectacles or surgery for ptosis. Since the cause is unknown, there is no specific medication for this disorder.

MYASTHENIA GRAVIS

Myasthenia gravis is a chronic disease causing fatigue of muscle groups; it has a predilection to first affect the ocular muscles before spreading to the other muscle masses. Palsy of various extraocular muscles is the usual presenting symptom, and the levator muscle is usually the first muscle involved. The easy fatigability of the muscle is manifest by an enhancement of the muscle palsy which is evident on forced use and also associated with general body fatigue. This causes a diurnal variation with the ptosis and muscle palsies being minimal or nonexistent in the morning and increasing as the day proceeds. Any type of strabismus may appear which is everchanging and almost impossible to accurately assess. However, weaknesses of convergence and upgaze are more common than any other gaze palsies. The inferior rectus muscle is commonly palsied intermittently, and this is unusual as an isolated entity. The lateral rectus muscle also is frequently palsied, and this may first be considered to be sixth nerve palsy rather than the true diagnosis of myasthenia gravis.

The onset of the ptosis or extraocular muscle involvement may occur at any age, even during infancy. The ophthalmologist is usually the first medical examiner having the opportunity to make this diagnosis. The ophthalmologist can easily fatigue the patient by demanding forceful, voluntary, rapid, repetitive version movement which cannot be sustained.

The electromyogram is diagnostic; as the muscle fatigues, action potentials begin to drop out to the point that the myogram becomes silent. The diagnosis is proved by injecting edrophonium bromide (Tensilon) or giving neostigmine either systemically or topically. Combining the administration of these drugs with the electromyography discloses an absolute improvement in the myogram; this increases the diagnostic capability because not invariably do these drugs totally eliminate the ptosis or strabismus, often giving an equivocal test response without the electromyogram.

The cause of myasthenia gravis is considered to be some curare type blocking effect of the acetylcholine at the myoneural junction. Since this is a systemic disease, the treatment of this disorder is outside the scope of ophthalmology and in the field of endocrinology. There are some poorly understood interrelationships in this disease between the thymus gland and the phenomenon of an autoimmunity reaction.

TRAUMA

Trauma is a common source of motility abnormality. The trauma may be produced by an external force disrupting the orbit, and it may be associated with damage to the extraocular muscles, causing strabismus. Trauma may also be produced by the surgeon operating either directly on the extraocular muscles or performing surgery for some other reason in their vicinity, eg, retinal detachment surgery. Probably one of the most traumatizing motility events that can occur is the surgeon either cutting the wrong muscle or losing a muscle.

ORBITAL FRACTURE

Orbital fractures may be caused by either direct trauma to the bones of the orbit or by blunt objects, larger than the diameter of the orbit, eg, a tennis ball, striking the eye with sufficient force to drive it back into the orbit, causing an intraorbital pressure wave that blows out the thin friable orbital bones. The blow-out fracture occurs in the floor, the medial wall, and the orbital roof where the orbital bones are paper thin. Blow-out fractures of the orbit are discussed with particular reference to their effect on ocular motility and the treatment for this disabling defect. The surgeon must always remember that more is involved in the fracture than simply a motility defect, and, until proved otherwise, intraocular injury and scleral rupture must always be suspected.

Blow-out fracture of the orbital floor is the commonest of the various orbital blow-out fractures. Immediately after the injury, ecchymosis of the lids appears and is associated with congestion of the orbital contents, causing proptosis. Pain is localized in the orbital floor, especially on vertical ocular movement attempts, particularly upgaze. Normal elevation and depression of the globe are restricted, and diplopia is noted. The vertical movements are most embarrassed with the eye in the abducted position if the inferior rectus muscle is the primary muscle involved in the fracture; however, with involvement of the inferior oblique muscle, the vertical movement may be interfered with both in adduction and in abduction. If the fracture site is near to or includes the infraorbital groove, the function of the infraorbital nerve is compromised; this causes either hypoesthesia or anesthesia over the lower eyelid, the cheek, and the lateral side of the nostril extending down to the upper lip.

The motility findings are varied according to the nature of the fracture, its size and location, and the specific tissue displaced and caught within the fracture site. The inferior oblique muscle and the inferior rectus muscle are either individually or both entrapped within the fracture. Depending on which muscle is entrapped, the extent of the entrapment determines whether in the primary position the eye is hypotropic, hypertropic, or neither; whether the restriction of ocular movement is greater in upgaze or in downgaze; and whether the restriction is equal in both adduction and in abduction or maximal in one vertical plane. The fracture may be a simple linear break without impingement of the orbital tissue or it may have hinged open long enough to catch tissue driven into it at the time of the initial impact, yet there is no bony defect apparent in the floor at the time of surgery. The fracture site may be a relatively large bony defect filled with orbital contents and spicules from the comminuted bones of the orbital floor. After the edema subsides, the initial proptosis may be replaced with enophthalmos if orbital tissue is incarcerated within the fracture site.

X-ray studies of the orbit and antrum should be obtained as soon as the patient's condition permits. Frequently, routine x-rays are negative despite an obvious floor fracture. A cloudy antrum is suggestive of trauma to the orbital floor, and the opaqueness is caused by accumulation of blood alone or blood plus orbital tissue within this space. Expertly performed tomography significantly increases the diagnostic localization of a floor fracture. A positive forced traction test performed with the patient either under topical or general anesthesia is usually helpful in differentiating the presence or absence of orbital contents impinged within a floor fracture, but it is not necessarily absolute. A patient known to have a floor fracture may have an equivocal traction test. Hemorrhage or edema within the muscle may cause transient paresis of the inferior rectus and inferior oblique muscles. Damage to the nerve entering the muscles or their myoneural junctions may cause the motility defect without impingement of the muscle or orbital content. This is usually transient with gradual improvement of the motility function during the first week to ten days following the injury, but, occasionally, the paresis produced by this method is permanent. Therefore, the motility defect may arise from the orbital trauma and have no relationship to the contiguous floor fracture.

Orbital medial wall fracture may be isolated or associated with floor or roof orbital fractures. The nasal orbital contents, including the medial rectus muscle, are usually incarcerated within the fracture of the laminae papyraceae. This causes considerable restriction of the horizontal ocular movements and also of the vertical movements to a limited degree. Tomograms and passive duction tests are helpful in the diagnosis, but, as with floor fractures, they are not invariably convincing.

Orbital roof fractures are associated with involvement of the levator and superior rectus muscles. Hence, ptosis and hypotropia are the usual findings along with an elevation restriction of the eye and maximal diplopia in upgaze.

Proper management of an orbital fracture demands first knowing whether or not the orbital contents are incarcerated within the fracture. Incarceration is an absolute indication for surgical exploration to correct this derangement of tissue. In addition to the motility considerations, enophthalmos can be prevented only by covering an obvious orbital defect with an alloplastic implant.

Occasionally the agony of making the decision to operate on a patient with persistent diplopia who is not improving within ten days following the injury can be frustrating. Conservative treatment directed at rapidly reducing the ecchymosis and edema, hoping to detect restoration of normal motility function, should be continued for the first ten days. If the motility defect does not improve by two weeks following trauma, surgery is usually indicated despite a negative tomogram, particularly if the traction test is positive. The best results occur from early liberation of the incarcerated tissue from the fracture. Only a small amount of orbital tissue needs to be caught in the fracture to interfere with motility. A small hinge fracture with only orbital fat caught is enough to interfere with normal motility. Fibrofatty proliferation results, and cicatrization gradually produces an increase in the eye alignment imbalance in the primary position. It is better to err on the side of early careful surgical investigation, finding nothing to explain the persistent motility defect, than to hope that the motility defect will disappear, only to learn that it does not as a result of impinged orbital tissue within the hinged fracture. The large blow-out fractures with obvious defects in the floor, medial wall, or roof are more definitely diagnosed by tomograms and clinical findings; hence, the torment confronting the ophthalmologist regarding the decision to operate is less.

Late repair of the orbital fracture is usually disappointing in regard to improving the motility defect. Investigation should still be attempted and a full assessment made before designing secondary surgery either on other muscles of the involved eye or of the contralateral eye. If ptosis and superior rectus muscle palsy are permanent residuals of an orbital roof fracture, surgery on the levator muscle and recession of the contralateral inferior oblique muscle is the best combination to improve this defect. These patients are usually near orthophoria in the primary position and have no defect in downgaze, so the surgeon does not wish to perform any surgery that puts these positions at risk. Therefore, recession of the direct antagonist of the paretic superior rectus muscle and resection of the paretic muscle should not be performed. Recession of the contralateral inferior oblique muscle improves the vertical movement in the position where it is needed, and it also improves the excyclodeviation associated with this condition.

SURGICAL TRAUMA

Surgical technique is important if surgery is to be performed without harm to the muscles, allowing for their reoperations several times if necessary. Vastly improved atraumatic surgical technique is available with newer sutures, fine needles, improved instrumentation, and refined techniques. The particular technique used should not place the conjunctival and Tenon's capsule incision directly over the surface of the muscle; it should displace the incision to the limbus or near the fornix, which avoids considerable scarring.

Direct visualization and identification of all muscles prior to cutting them is essential to prevent cutting the wrong muscle. For instance, blindly sweeping for the inferior oblique muscle between the lateral border of the inferior rectus muscle and the insertion of the inferior oblique muscle can result in the inferior rectus muscle or the lateral rectus muscle being cut either along with or instead of the inferior oblique muscle. The same danger prevails with the blind sweep for the superior oblique tendon where the superior rectus muscle can inadvertently be cut either instead of or along with the superior oblique tendon. Hence, fishing blindly with a muscle hook into the incisional area, hoping to pull up into the operative field the inferior oblique muscle or the superior oblique tendon, should be condemned. These muscles should always be approached by direct visualization, and techniques have been described to accomplish this (13, 14).

Surgery on the retina is not without trauma to the extraocular muscles, and placement of encircling bands and exoplants have distorted and traumatized muscles and produced motility defects. The superior oblique tendon is prone to be displaced forward to the nasal border of the insertion of the superior rectus muscle; this causes a kinked taut tendon resulting in incyclodeviation, hypotropia, limitation of elevation in adduction, and limitation of abduction.

Severance of the superior oblique tendon has occurred when the nasal horn of the levator muscle is blindly cut during the levator resection for ptosis. Creation of massive adhesions between the superior rectus and the levator muscles during surgery on the levator has also produced vertical deviations and elevation deficiency. The inverse of this problem is for ptosis to result from massive orbital hemorrhage caused by blindly sweeping for the superior oblique tendon or traumatic surgery on the superior rectus muscle.

Traumatizing the neatly compartmented orbital fat pad which is arranged peripheral to the muscle cone, allowing the fat to mix with blood in the operative field, forms fibrofatty proliferation that attaches to the external muscles and sclera; this causes unanticipated embarrassment of motility. The fibrofatty proliferation undergoes cicatrization, forming taut bands causing a deviation of the eye which gradually increases with time, restricting the movement of the eye as it attempts to move in the direction opposite to the bands. The surgeon should make every effort to prevent traumatizing the orbital fat pads during extraocular surgery.

LOST MUSCLES

The lost muscle is usually the medial rectus muscle and frequently occurs during a resection procedure. It is difficult to lose the other three rectus muscles because of their connection to the oblique muscles. The superior rectus muscle is attached to the superior oblique tendon sheath, and, hence, it does not recoil back into the orbit when it is inadvertently cut. The lateral rectus and inferior rectus muscles are also attached to the inferior oblique muscle, and this locks them in a forward position where they can readily be found if cut. These rectus muscles coil into a small mass at the site of attachment to the respective obliques, but they can be uncoiled and brought forward and attached to the original insertion sites. However,

since the medial rectus muscle has no attachment to any other muscle, it snaps back through Tenon's capsule at the point it enters, as it proceeds from the origin to the insertion, making it almost impossible for the surgeon to find. However, if this is recognized at the time of surgery, a diligent prolonged search, using wide exposure and a Desmarres lid retractor to spread the tissues apart, is the only chance of ever finding the muscle. The best source of illumination for working in this deep hole is the indirect ophthalmoscope which the surgeon should place on his head before proceeding with the tedious search. If the medial rectus muscle cannot be found, it is a mistake to bring Tenon's tissue up and attach it to the insertion site of the medial rectus muscle since this creates severe limitations of horizontal and vertical ductions. The better solution for this disastrous motility problem is transposition of the nasal halves of the superior and inferior rectus muscles to the insertion site of the medial rectus muscle.

Diagnosis of the lost muscle late after it occurred at surgery is not easy, although one sign is helpful: as the eye attempts to move into the field of action of the lost muscle, it protrudes and the palpebral fissure widens. This is due to the relaxation of the ipsilateral antagonist and the absence of an intact opponent rectus muscle, reducing the retraction effect that the rectus muscles exert on the eye. Whenever the diagnosis is made, the surgical exploration designed to correct the motility defect should proceed forthrightly.

REFERENCES

1. Brown HW: In Allen JH (ed): Strabismus Ophthalmic Symposium I. St. Louis: Mosby, 1950, p 205
2. Huber A: Duane's retraction syndrome: Considerations on pathogenesis and aetiology of the different forms of Duane's retraction syndrome. In Strabismus. St. Louis: Mosby, 1969, p 36
3. Kirkham TH: Inheritance of Duane's syndrome. Br J Ophthalmol 54:323, 1970
4. Pfaffenbach DD, Cross HE, Kearns TP: Congenital anomalies in Duane's retraction syndrome. Arch Ophthalmol 88:635, 1972
5. Wildervanck LS: Een cervico-oculo-acusticus-syndroom. Ned Tijdschr Geneeskd 104:2600, 1960
6. Breinin GM: Electromyography—A tool in ocular and neurologic diagnosis. Arch Ophthalmol 57:165, 1957
7. Blodi FC, van Allen MW, Yarbrough JC: Duane's syndrome: A Brain Stem Lesion. Arch Ophthalmol 72:171, 1964
8. Brown HW: Isolated inferior oblique paralysis: An analysis of 97 cases. Trans Am Ophthalmol Soc 55:415, 1957
9. Brown HW: In Haik GM (ed): Strabismus Symposium of the New Orleans Academy of Ophthalmology. St. Louis: Mosby, 1962

10. Brown HW: True and simulated superior oblique tendon sheath syndromes. Doc Ophthalmol 34:123, 1973

11. Scott AB, Knapp P: Surgical treatment of the superior oblique tendon sheath syndrome. Arch Ophthalmol 88:282, 1972

12. Khodadoust AA, von Noorden GK: Bilateral vertical retraction syndrome. Arch Ophthalmol 78:606, 1967

13. Parks MM, Helveston EM: Direct visualization of the superior oblique tendon. Arch Ophthalmol 84:491, 1970

14. Parks MM: A study of the weakening surgical procedures for eliminating overaction of the inferior oblique muscle. Trans Am Ophthalmol Soc 69:163, 1971; Am J Ophthalmol 73:107, 1972

Index

Cover and text designed by M. S. Karkucinski

Composition by American Book, Stratford Press
Printing by Murray Printing, Inc.

Harper & Row, Publishers

75 76 77 78 79 80   10 9 8 7 6 5 4 3 2 1